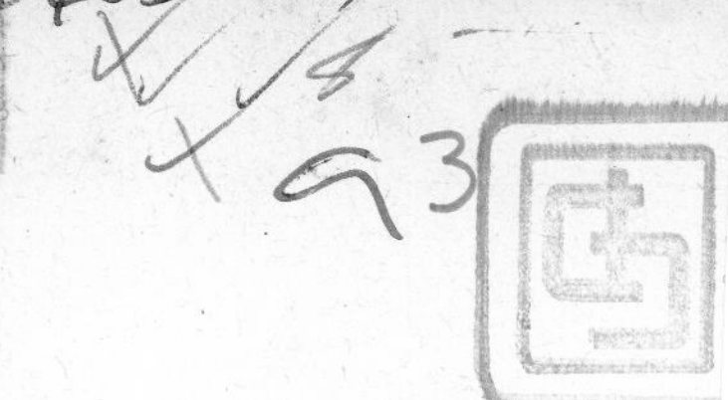

WATER

Solutions to a Problem of Supply and Demand

REVISED EDITION

Michael Overman

The Open University Press

Designer: **Arthur Lockwood**
Research: **Joy Jacques**
Diagrams: **John Messenger, David Nash, Gillian Newing, and Edward Poulton**

The Open University Press
A division of
Open University Educational Enterprises Limited
12 Cofferidge Close
Milton Keynes MK11 1BY, England

First published 1968 in the United Kingdom by Aldus Books Limited.
First published in this revised edition 1976 by The Open University Press

Reprinted 1981

Printed and bound in Great Britain
by Billing and Sons Limited,
Guildford, London, Oxford, Worcester.

ISBN 0 335 00046 0

Contents

Water measurement

1 cubic meter (1 m^3)	=	220 Imperial gallons
	=	264 U.S. gallons
4500 m^3	=	1 million Imperial gallons
3788 m^3	=	1 million U.S. gallons

Author's Note to this Edition

When this book was written it was intended for the general reader who might have no scientific knowledge while being interested in the impact of technology on contemporary life. When the book was chosen as required reading in the Open University course *Environmental Control and Public Health*, it became desirable to expand and clarify a few passages in the text and it seemed appropriate that this should be done by Dr Andrew Porteous, who was responsible for preparation of the course material. Accordingly this edition includes a series of short notes compiled by Dr Porteous. These notes not only give the reader useful new information but bring the book up-to-date.

Dr Porteous and I also thought that a new edition should include a short additional chapter on "Water Resources Planning", a discipline which has assumed enormous importance in recent years in many areas where the rainfall is low in relation to the growing population. The new material is now included as a postscript, and I would like to thank Sir M. MacDonald & Partners, consulting engineers of Cambridge, who specialize in the engineering of water, for supplying me with much up-to-date information.

1 June 1976
Walkern, Herts.

Michael Overman

SAVE WATER

1 Toward a Crisis

The thirst of civilized man is insatiable. The more sophisticated he becomes the thirstier he seems to grow. In the so-called developing countries as little as 12 liters of fresh water sometimes suffices as the daily supply for each person, while in London domestic consumption exceeds 150 liters per head every 24 hours. Even this figure is surpassed by the demand in the more prosperous cities of the United States, where 250 liters per head is typical of the daily domestic demand in urban areas. Yet this is only part of the story; for as man becomes more advanced he needs more and more water for commerce, industry, public institutions like hotels and hospitals, power stations, and many other uses. Add to this unremitting increase in demand the ceaseless growth in the world's population, and we have a glimpse of the extent of the problem it presents, a problem that today seems to be moving slowly but inexorably toward a crisis in more and more areas around the world.

A water crisis in New York. Low rainfall during the previous four years coupled with mismanagement and wastage of existing water supplies produced, in the summer of 1965, the worst drought on record. The Hudson River, polluted by industrial and domestic waste, flowed untapped through the city.

Supply and Demand

Why should this be so when water is the most plentiful of all natural substances? In short, the problem is one of matching supply with demand. For example, in the summer of 1965 the reservoirs supplying water to New York City were on the point of completely drying up. Ironically, the Hudson River, which flows through the city, could not be used as a water supply because of heavy domestic and industrial pollution. Nor is New York unique among cities. In great conurbations all over the world, providing adequate water supply in all seasons is an unresolved problem; in Calcutta, which like New York stands astride a great river, it is a problem that has been described as a municipal nightmare.

If the growth of domestic and industrial demand for water has been taxing the ability of management to meet it, how does agriculture fare? It has been estimated that a man weighing 75 kilograms requires 750 kg. of water a year. But to grow 75 kg. of wheat needs well over 100,000 kg. of water—such is the thirst of vegetable matter. As the world's population rises, so must food production increase, and as the farmer strives to produce more food from his land, he must clearly use more and more water. In agriculture, as in industry, there are numerous locations where a real problem exists. Yet here we find, all too often, an anomaly that bears an unhappy resemblance to the 1965 plight of New York—the existence, often side by side, of vast potential supplies of water and immense tracts of potentially fertile land rendered impotent through lack of rain. Africa possesses some 40 per cent of the earth's running fresh water and millions of square kilometers of fertile land; yet Africa produces only 2 per cent of the world's food.

Africa is so underpopulated that it has only experienced a major water problem in the extreme north—in Egypt, Tunisia, Morocco, and Algeria. How different from India and Pakistan, where agriculture, vital to the lives of millions of people, suffers regular setbacks: uncontrolled floods during the monsoon rains—floods that destroy thousands of square kilometers of summer food crops; and failure of the winter rains, irrevocably stunting the northern wheat crop. In a relatively small continent with an alarmingly large population this spells famine year after year. Yet northern India and Pakistan are excellently endowed with water. The Indus River alone is one of the world's greatest natural sources of fresh water. Together with its five tributaries, the Indus carries more than twice the average annual flow of the Nile. As much as half of this water is diverted to feed the world's most highly developed system of irrigation canals; but the rest—equal to the mighty Nile's entire flow—runs to waste. True, the flow of the Indus and its tributaries varies with the season. In midsummer, when water is most needed, it is reduced to little more than a trickle. But even total failure of the rains in northern India ought not to spell catastrophe, for under the Indus basin lies a vast subterranean reservoir, the porous rock of which holds at least 10 times the total annual flow of the river. Yet poverty and hunger persist. The same story can be told of eastern India, where millions of peasant farmers live in even greater poverty than those in the northwest, suffering drought, and therefore famine, year after year. Yet the Ganges and Brahmaputra rivers together carry millions of cubic meters of water annually into the Bay of Bengal, often flooding huge areas of the countryside in the process.

Israel is a country in which most of the water for agricultural, domestic, and industrial use has had to be obtained from under the ground; there is no other source. This was extremely promising 25 years ago, for there appeared to be plenty, which only needed pumping out. But in the early 1950s, when demand was steadily rising, it was noticed that the output of the natural springs was dropping; the uncomfortable inference was that reserves had fallen below the safe limit. Water was available in quantities in Lake Tiberias (the biblical Sea of Galilee) in the extreme north of Israel, but the demand was mainly in the south, over 150 km. away. In so dry a country, where the surface sand dunes can soak up immeasurable quantities of water, a canal to bring the water south would have had to be waterproofed throughout—an extremely costly expedient. This fact and the inevitable losses by evaporation on the way would have rendered the water that reached the southern farmlands too expensive for the economic production of fruit. Here was a water problem that was solved in an ingenious way. Israel's subterranean water-bearing rocks lie in a continuous layer from north to south. So Israeli engineers tried pumping water out of Lake Tiberias into the depleted wells in the north. As they had hoped, this added water began slowly to replenish the underground reserves and in due course the fallen water level in wells in the far south began to rise. The *aquifer*, as the underground water-bearing rock layer is called, was being used as a natural conduit, costing nothing to build; and, being underground, there was no loss by evaporation. Today Israel consumes far more water than she did a decade ago. However, a new problem looms ahead. The water consumption curve goes relentlessly up and the aquifer's capacity to convey water southward will one day prove inadequate. Water supply pipelines of various diameters have been in operation as part of Israel's national distribution system since the 1930s, but only recently have large-diameter sections come into use. Most notable of these is the National Water Carrier, a concrete pipeline 3 m. in diameter and 130 km. long, which diverts 320 million cubic meters (Mm^3) of water annually from Lake Tiberias in the north to Rosh Ha'ayin in central Israel. From here further pipelines convey the water to the potentially fertile land of the Negev region in the south. However, using all available water resources, only 40 per cent of Israel's irrigable land can be adequately supplied. Seawater desalination plants are already in operation in places where their application is economic, such as Elath in the southern Negev. As outlined in the final chapter, large-scale desalination of the sea might well be the most realistic solution to Israel's local water shortage problem.

Consider Kuwait, that tiny barren sheikhdom of hot sun and sand on the shores of the Persian Gulf. This little country has no natural supply of fresh water other than rain, of which a paltry 10 cm. falls each year during the monsoon season. When oil was discovered and gold began to flow, the oil companies required more and more men to live there. The local Arabs had conditioned themselves to an almost waterless existence, but the newcomers could not work without it. So when enterprising sailors found that the oil men could pay any price for water they began to trade in it, bringing it in kegs down the coast by boat from the nearest river, 100 km. to the north. In Kuwait's capital they sold it, literally, to the thirsty men of business. But soon the oil men decided it was time to find themselves cheaper water. In 1950 the Kuwait Oil Company financed the country's first desalination plant, producing 3000 m^3 of fresh water daily from the sea—over seven times Kuwait's previous daily consumption. The company installed the plant for its own private

The National Water Carrier in Israel. Completed in 1967, this is a major link in a series of schemes to improve local distribution of irrigation water and to supply the arid Negev region of the south with water from Lake Tiberias in northern Israel. From the Eshed Kinrot pumping station (A) water flows 130 km.—by way of tunnel, canal, and 3-m-diameter concrete pipeline—to Rosh Ha'ayin (B) in central Israel. With additional supply from the Yarkon River, the water continues in a dual pipeline system of about 2-m. diameter and then, by way of small-bore local conduits, to Beersheba and the central Negev. Frontiers are pre-1967. Below: laying 3-m. pipeline.

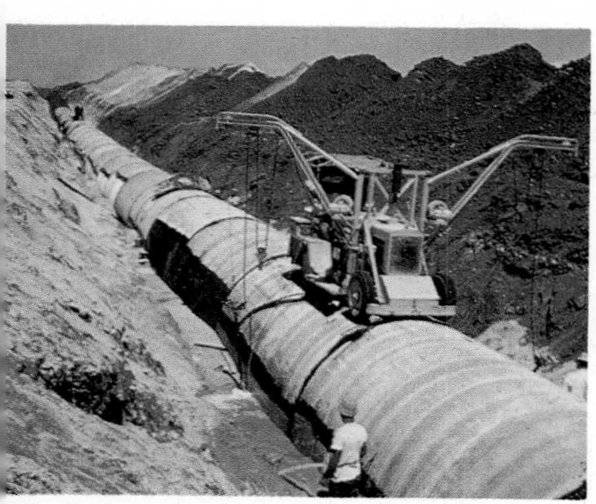

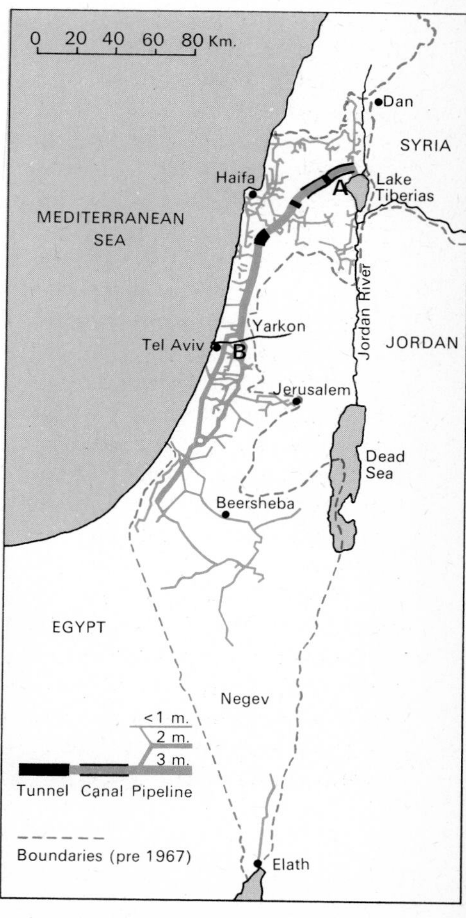

use, but within a year the government had negotiated to purchase for public use some of the water produced. The government soon realized that desalination provided an answer to its immediate water problem, and commissioned a plant of its own. By March 1953 this new plant began to supply the city with 5000 m^3 of distilled seawater each day. Subsequently, with demand ever rising, further plants were installed, in 1955, 1957, and 1960, and subsequent additions have raised the total installed capacity to 87,600 m^3/day. So Kuwait, once a desert encampment, is today not only an oil-rich city, but a city with more than adequate water; it even has a limited but flourishing agriculture specializing in the production of vegetables and poultry. Of course water in Kuwait is expensive; but this is no problem since Kuwait can afford to buy it with oil. Nor is the government content with the present position. The latest plan, by agreement with Iraq, is to build a pipeline carrying excess river water from Basra—a pipeline capable of transporting what to a Kuwait of 20 years ago would represent a veritable flood—600,000 m^3 of water a day.

Desalination, as a means of increasing fresh-water supply, is only made use of in situations where conventional water engineering methods cannot be employed. Dams, reservoirs, and river diversion schemes are in operation in many countries of the world.

The Aswan High Dam is one eloquent example. Here is a single dam capable of holding back more than the entire annual flow of the Nile. In southeast Australia, too, we can see the remarkable Snowy Mountain project, by which engineers have diverted, across a mountain ridge, an annual 3000 Mm^3 of water. This water originally flowed eastward through country adequately endowed with rainfall (where the river water was consequently of little value), but it has now been diverted into westward-flowing rivers that pass through dry but fertile plains. The resulting increase in crop production has been valued at some $90 million a year.

The southwestern states of the United States include a huge region that is generally short of water, where the further development of agriculture is already in jeopardy. The current average annual demand for water in this region has been estimated at 90,000 Mm^3. To meet this demand underground supplies have been exploited for many years; but the wells are now drying up. Water has been pumped out faster than nature can replenish it. If agriculture continues to develop at the rate of recent years, the annual demand will increase by over 45 per cent during the next quarter century. But with water running short already, where can the extra come from? Neighboring areas to the northeast have a surplus of water and could supply the deficit. But to transport the 40,000 Mm^3 of water needed would cost about $3000 million a year, or $7\frac{1}{2}$ cents/m^3. A University of New Mexico study has estimated that the economy of the American Southwest profits by between 3.6 and 4.25 cents/m^3 of water used in irrigation—substantially less than the cost of bringing water in from the north. The same study has shown, however, that the development of industry in this region brings in a profit of between \$2.50/m^3 and \$3.35/m^3 of water utilized. This pinpoints one of the crucial facts of water management. The problem here in the Southwest can be resolved by putting up the price of water and, in order to meet it, by shifting the emphasis of the economy from agriculture to industry. Up to a point this is all very well; but in a world of ever-increasing population any reduction in the area producing food must be matched by a corresponding increase elsewhere. To solve a water crisis by precipitating one of food is clearly no solution.

The paradox I have described in these pages may be restated very simply. Ample water exists in our world for all man's needs; but much of it is either in the wrong place or in the wrong form. If the problem were as simple as that, there would be no cause for concern. Unfortunately it is a highly complex state of affairs, which, until comparatively recent times, man has neglected to study. Suddenly, when water runs short, he finds it is a problem that takes time to solve. In the meantime demand continues to grow and the question becomes one not so much of meeting tomorrow's requirements, as of catching up with the past. This is beginning to apply in water-short regions the world over, and unless decisive action is taken wherever demand is overreaching supply, man will find himself on the threshold not of a problem, but of a crisis. If such a crisis threatens it is fortunately one of management, not of technology. Once authority takes the right decisions, science will not be wanting. Hydrologists, chemists, bacteriologists, and engineers between them know how the paradox can be turned around to man's advantage. The hydrologist knows where water is to be found; the chemist and bacteriologist, how to purify it; the engineer can deliver it where and when it is wanted.

It is the engineer who plays the spectacular role. Once the hydrologist has located the source of supply, he is forgotten. The part played by the chemist and bacteriologist is vital to health, yet is rarely noticed until a water treatment plant fails in its job. The great dam, the supply canal, the mountain aqueduct, stands witness to the engineer's skill. Yet not one of these experts alone can quench man's thirst. Together they work to harness great rivers, to find and pump water from under the ground, to cleanse it of impurities, to remove, if need be, even the salt from the sea.

The engineering of water is expensive. Large dams, among the most expensive of all civil engineering works, often involve their sponsors in immense social and political problems that must be solved before the engineer can get to work. Despite the troubles they sometimes cause, and despite their awe-inspiring cost, dams have a great redeeming feature. Not only do they divert millions of cubic meters of water to the thirsty plains, but they provide man with the opportunity to convert the unending energy of that water's movement into useful power. Hydroelectric power will never, by itself, solve man's power supply problem, but, unlike the power produced from the world's dwindling resources of coal, oil, natural gas (and now even uranium), water power will never dry up as long as nature supports life. The concrete of the dams is as likely to crumble first.

Man's Water Requirement

Before we can begin to analyze man's water supply problem we must not only know what he uses today, but estimate what he is likely to use tomorrow. It is extremely difficult to make realistic estimates of the world's current usage of water, let alone its future requirement. Statistics are hopelessly incomplete and, when it comes to forecasting, there are too many uncertain variables. If the figures that follow are estimates based, in some cases, on other estimates, they should nevertheless serve to give the reader an indication of the immensity of the problem.

The average daily consumption of water in a large modern city is sometimes as much as 2000 liters per head, a figure that includes commercial, industrial, and public consumption. A

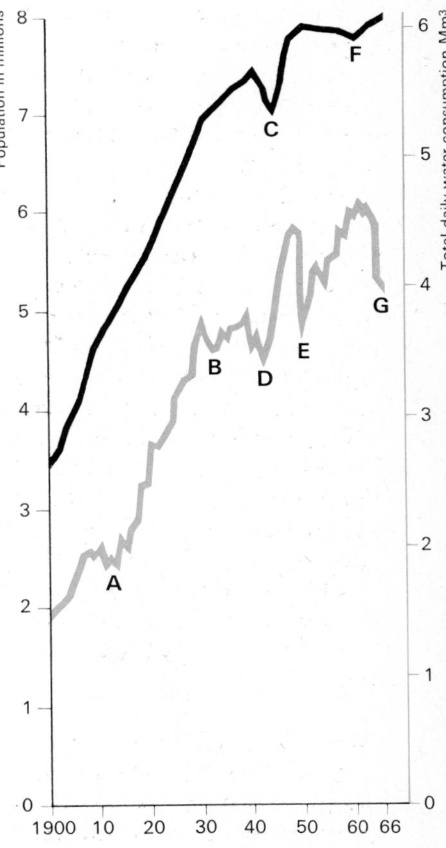

The population curve (black) and total water consumption curve (blue) for New York City from 1900 illustrate the increase in water demand typical of many large cities in the world. The letters refer to deviations from steady increase curves. (A) Conservation measures necessary before the introduction of a new water supply source. (B) Conservation during water shortage. (C) Population shift into armed forces and outside industries during World War II. (D) Reduction in consumption during wartime and restrictions following drought in 1941. (E) Intensive conservation following serious drought in 1949. (F) Population shift into the suburbs. (G) The severe drought of 1965, in which normal consumption was reduced by 20 per cent.

more typical figure for the average city is 500 liters per head per day. Against this, a castaway on an arid, uninhabited island might live on about one liter a day, though his life would be considerably more comfortable with five. Some primitive tribes probably manage with five liters per head per day during periods of natural shortage.

Clearly we are already in trouble if we are to forecast future trends. The most competent statistician would find it hard to justify an "average" daily consumption anywhere between these extremes. Statistics do show, however, that urban water consumption (including industrial demand) is increasing at a steady rate of approximately one per cent per head per year.

In the United States, where the population is expected to grow by 35 million between 1970 and 1980, an increase in urban water demand of one per cent per head per year would result in a total increase of almost 30 per cent over the 10-year period. This would be subdivided into: 16 per cent for population growth at the current demand rate; 11 per cent for demand increase of the original population; and 2 per cent for demand increase of the additional population. So for all the average-sized water supply stations in the United States today (commissioned during the past 100 years), the need may arise to establish one third as many more in the 10 years to come. This is, of course, an oversimplification of the facts, but it is intended to serve as a pointer to the order of the problem faced by planners and engineers. The pointer is no exaggeration.

Urban supply does not end with the dam, the groundwater pumping station, or the desalination plant. It also involves the problem of transporting, purifying, storing locally, and distributing the water; and, ultimately, of disposing of it when it reappears, polluted. Thus, a demand increase of 30 per cent in 10 years involves, not only a 30-per-cent increase in primary supply, but an equivalent increase in the capacity of supply mains, purification plants, local storage and distributing systems, city sewers, and sewage treatment plants. Growing urban demand presents a special problem, since not only does the increased supply of water have to be collected from farther and farther afield as existing sources fall short of demand, but all this water has to be channeled into a restricted area that is growing ever more congested.

I mentioned earlier that urban demand includes domestic, communal, commercial, and industrial requirements. In fact, while domestic consumption (for sanitation, cleaning, cooking, and household gardening) accounts for about 45 per cent of the total amount used in a typical modern city, commerce and industry consume about as much again, the balance (10 per cent) being accounted for by public institutions and services.

For all I have said so far, urban water demand is, in fact, only a small part of man's total requirement, which necessarily includes the water needed to supply him with food. Fortunately, this is not so immense a problem as the world's population explosion statistics would seem to indicate. Natural rainfall still provides the bulk of the water needed by crops in large areas of the world. In parts of India, and in Egypt and the Middle East generally, where industrial production is insufficient to provide the means for the purchase of food from areas hydrologically better endowed, the availability of water on the land is a positive regulator of life. It is significant to note that in Egypt the increasing volume of Nile water brought under control since the turn of the century corelates unmistakably with the rising population curve.

On a worldwide scale agricultural water consumption is immense. Ten per cent of the world's total land area—some 1250 million hectares (1 hectare is 10,000 m^2)—are cultivated, one per cent of this being under man-made irrigation. This irrigated one per cent utilizes about $1\frac{1}{2}$ Mm^3 of water each year. The remainder is watered by rainfall and underground seepage totaling a further $13\frac{1}{2}$ million Mm^3 of water. One acre-foot (the traditional Imperial unit for the measurement of agricultural water) is approximately equal to 1234 m^3.

Consider the humble cabbage. This, like any other plant, obtains a part of its food by a process that involves the absorption of water from the soil by its roots, the passage of that water up its stem and into its leaves, and its evaporation from the leaf pores into the atmosphere, a process termed *transpiration.* A typical cabbage, in the act of growing from seed to full size, transpires some 25 kg. of water. To grow a kilogram of wheat requires 1500 kg. of water. The same quantity of rice requires nearly three times as much water. Turning to cash crops, we find that production of a kilogram of cotton involves the transpiration of no less than 10,000 kg. of water. Where meat is concerned, we must supply water both for growing the animal's food and for the animal itself. To produce a single egg, for example, requires about 1000 kg. of water.

Man needs water for his crops and his own life processes, but with the present rate of technological development, water used in industry is occupying an ever-increasing part of man's total water requirement. Water can dissolve a larger number of substances, in greater amounts, than any other solvent. It is this property that makes it, cheap as it is, so important in the chemical industry for both conveying raw materials in solution, and washing away waste products. The man in the street is

The table illustrates the quantity of water consumed in the production of 1 kg. of common agricultural and industrial commodities. The high consumption figure for 1 kg. of eggs includes the water transpired during growth of the animal's food as well as that used in the animal's own growth processes. In industry, water is used for washing, cooling, and conveyance of substances in solution or suspension.

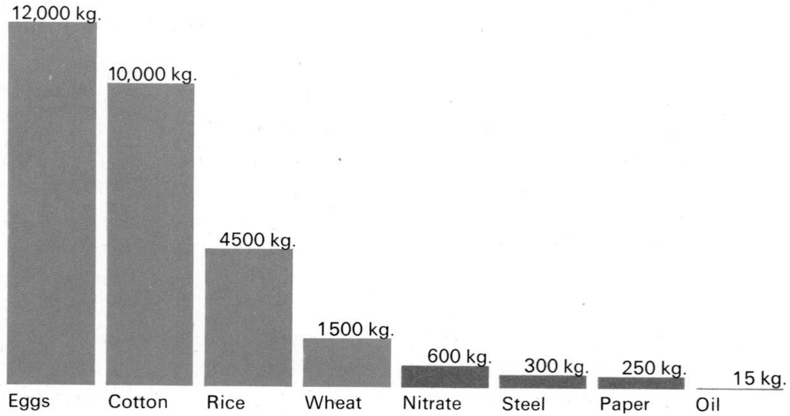

often astonished to learn how much water is "consumed" by industry. Typical figures are 300 kg. of water for every kilogram of steel manufactured, 250 kg. for every kilogram of paper, and 600 kg. for every kilogram of nitrate fertilizer. Such water is used for washing, cooling, and the conveyance of other substances (partly in solution, partly in suspension) and most of it emerges from the factory polluted, often seriously.

Water is widely used in industry to convey heat. Water has a high *specific heat*—i.e. to raise the temperature of a given quantity of water by a given number of degrees requires a greater amount of heat than would be needed by most other substances. For example, nearly six times as much heat is required to bring water to a given temperature as is needed for the equivalent amount of air. When water vapor condenses and hot water cools, the stored heat energy is released. This explains the value of water and of steam as media for the transfer of heat in industry: in heat exchangers; for the conversion of heat into mechanical energy; and as a general coolant.

This property, whereby water and its vapor can store and convey relatively large quantities of heat, is made the more useful by the ease with which it can be piped from one location to another. So useful is this facility that in most American and Soviet nuclear reactors water is used as the medium to convey heat from the core to the heat exchangers, where steam to drive the turbine generators is produced. Water is also used as a *moderator* in water-cooled reactors. A moderator slows down neutrons (uncharged atomic particles emitted by uranium) to the optimum speed required to produce fission in another uranium atom. The disadvantage is that water absorbs a high percentage of neutrons and is only effective with enriched uranium. "Heavy water" (composed of the hydrogen isotope deuterium) is a good moderator and absorbs hardly any neutrons. It is, however, expensive to produce.

The Problem of Wasted Water

Everywhere we look we can see water running to waste. Survey analysis has demonstrated conclusively that the provision of water meters for individual consumers, and charging according to consumption, is the surest method of minimizing domestic wastage. One sample survey, which covered 136 American towns and cities with populations exceeding 25,000, showed that the daily consumption per head worked out at 650 liters where less than 10 per cent of supplies were metered, but was only 265 liters in areas where 50 per cent or more houses had meters.

There is undoubtedly scope for very considerable reduction of wastage in both domestic and industrial water usage, but far more significant as a solution to the imbalance of world resources is a reduction of waste in agriculture. About half the very considerable volume of water provided through engineering for crop irritation is lost before it reaches the field. Less than half the water that does reach the field is actually used in the life process of plants. Exactly what steps may be taken to effect maximum savings is largely a matter of conjecture, for it is an area in which research is urgently required.

Obviously losses from water channels by seepage can be avoided, or at least reduced, by suitably lining the channels, but existing methods may be too expensive to justify their adoption, because the price of the harvest would be beyond the currently economic limit. Research might develop cheap means of rendering water channels impervious, perhaps by some one-pass soil-stabilization and waterproofing process. This could also inhibit the growth of water-loving weeds.

Losses by evaporation from the soil surface, if not wholly avoidable, can be substantially reduced by new mulching methods (covering the soil—traditionally with a layer of compost or sawdust). The application of a microscopically fine film of cetyl alcohol to the surface of large reservoirs is being used in warm countries to reduce surface evaporation. This compound, which is nontoxic and invisible to the naked eye when it is spread on water, controls evaporation while permitting the passage of oxygen and sunlight—both essential to the natural self-purification process—and also of rain. Perhaps this or a similar process can be applied to slow-moving water in channels. Perhaps even the water requirements of the crops themselves can be modified so that either the ratio of yield to transpiration may be raised, or species tolerant to salty water developed. In Israel, work in this latter direction has already met with some success, and crops have been grown that accept irrigation by salt-laden water. This saves on the fresh water that would otherwise have to be flushed through the land to leach out the salt lethal to conventional crops (see Chapter 4).

The Water Paradox

I opened this chapter with the presentation of a simple but uncomfortable fact: that though ample water exists in our world, man is failing to deliver it where it is wanted. It is little short of criminal negligence that, in a world well-endowed with water, man is failing to satisfy the hunger of millions (for

Water losses in irrigation. Evaporation rate from the surface of water in the reservoir (A) depends on temperature, humidity, and wind speed. A "no loss" concrete pipe (B) conveys water to a concrete-lined main distribution channel (C). Here evaporation also occurs. Sloping earth channels (D) direct the water onto the fields (E). Seepage and escape from (D) and seepage below the root zone at (E) together represent 50 per cent of all irrigation water losses. The upward arrows from (E) indicate water loss by evaporation from the soil plus transpiration by the crops (i.e. evaporation of water already used in growth processes). Excess water runs off as streams (F).

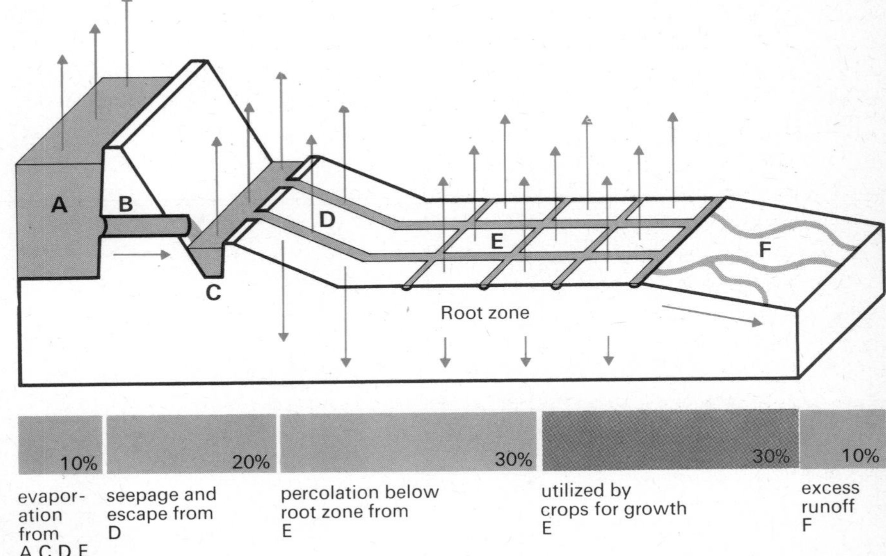

example in India) or to quench the agricultural and industrial thirst of millions more (as in the southwest United States).

The inescapable inference to which the admittedly incomplete information leads is that a water crisis is creeping up and may overtake the advance of civilized man. The anomaly lies in the fact that the crisis that threatens our era of technical knowledge is the product of ignorance and apathy, sheltered in some cases, under the umbrella of ethics.

Technically man is perfectly capable of supplying the total demand for agricultural, industrial, and domestic fresh water. Moreover, man's total foreseeable requirement in the next 1000 years is, quite literally, a drop in the ocean: not more than one per cent of the water in the sea. Large-scale desalination is an important possibility. It can be undertaken with the aid of nuclear power with virtually no fuel transport, smoke, or waste-product riddles to be solved, and no other problem than the existing one of moving the end product to the point of consumption. So conscious is the United States of the potential importance of desalination that in the 1967 financial year the government set aside no less than $91 million for research and development in this field.

However, desalination is by no means the most important way of obtaining supplies of water. As we shall see in Chapter 2, natural evaporation from the surface of the oceans exceeds precipitation into the sea by approximately 9 per cent. This 9 per cent falls on the land and runs back to the sea mostly in the form of rivers. It is 9 per cent of a very large quantity, representing an annual freshwater flow, distilled for free by the sun, adding up to some 40 million Mm^3. This alone is more than man's annual need.

Then, too, there are vast reserves of water below the surface of the earth. The quantity within the top three-quarter kilometer is estimated currently at some 5000 million Mm^3. Some of this is locked so deep in or under rock that we must discount it, but there is plenty that can be pumped out by accepted engineering methods. Why then does contemporary engineering and water management sometimes fail to meet man's needs? The root of the problem is that from the beginning of time water has been counted as a gift of nature. Traditionally it has been free because, as rain, it could be collected in its pure form by anyone who cared to run a pipe from the gutters of his house to a water butt; and because, as river water, it could be lifted out by anyone with a bucket. Unlike the majority of nature's gifts there was no processing, no factory involved until man began to pollute nature's supply more rapidly than nature could purify it. If we have to pay a water rate today it is chiefly a handling and purification charge. In the United States this amounts to one per cent of the gross national product and water costs, on the average, one cent per cubic meter. This is a fair price to pay for water—or so thinks John Citizen—especially when the purification necessary is, as we have said, almost invariably the result of pollution caused by man himself.

If water were provided by big business on a supply-and-demand basis, a very different picture would emerge. Like gasoline ($13/m^3$) or milk ($60) or whisky ($600 plus tax), it would be supplied where and when it was wanted in whatever

Livestock farmers water their animals at a well hole in western India. Underground water reservoirs (aquifers) are the only available source of water in such arid regions, where evaporation of surface water occurs rapidly.

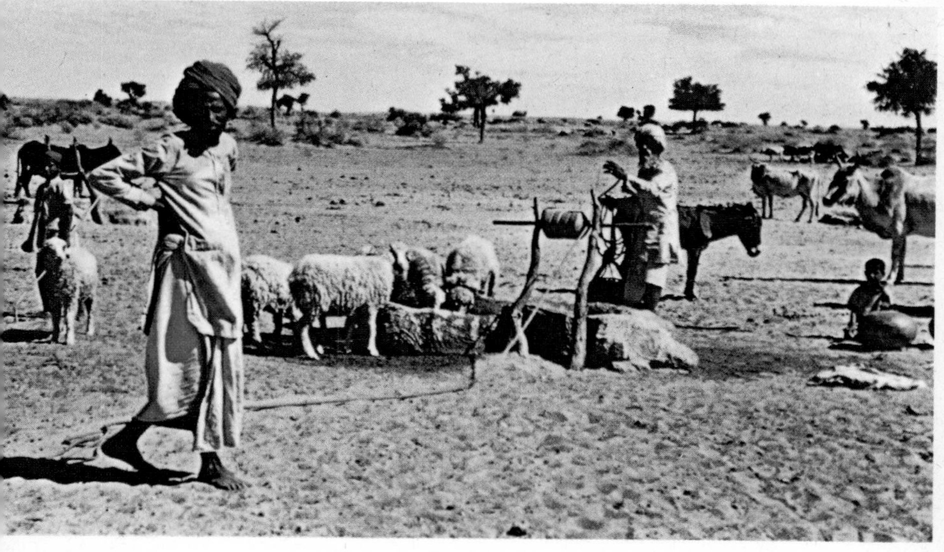

quantity required. The price would be related to the capital and running costs of the engineering required to gather, purify, and deliver it. There would be no shortage in New York for those who were willing to pay the price.

That the economics of water supply is far more complex than the average educated man is accustomed to believe is illustrated by the findings I have already quoted of a University of New Mexico research project. This study investigated the value added to the economy of southwestern states when water supplies were increased. Irrigation agriculture was shown to boost the economy of the area studied by approximately 4 cents/m^3 supplied, whereas water supplied to industry benefited the economy by not less than \$2.50/m^3. If water supplies can be augmented in this area at a cost above the U.S. average, who is to fix the price? If industry is prepared to buy water at a price the farmer cannot afford and the domestic consumer considers unfair, does this mean that industry must

The aim of water engineering schemes is to match supply with demand. Flooding, here of the Godavari River in western India, represents water running to waste that could be impounded and used to irrigate dry-season crops.

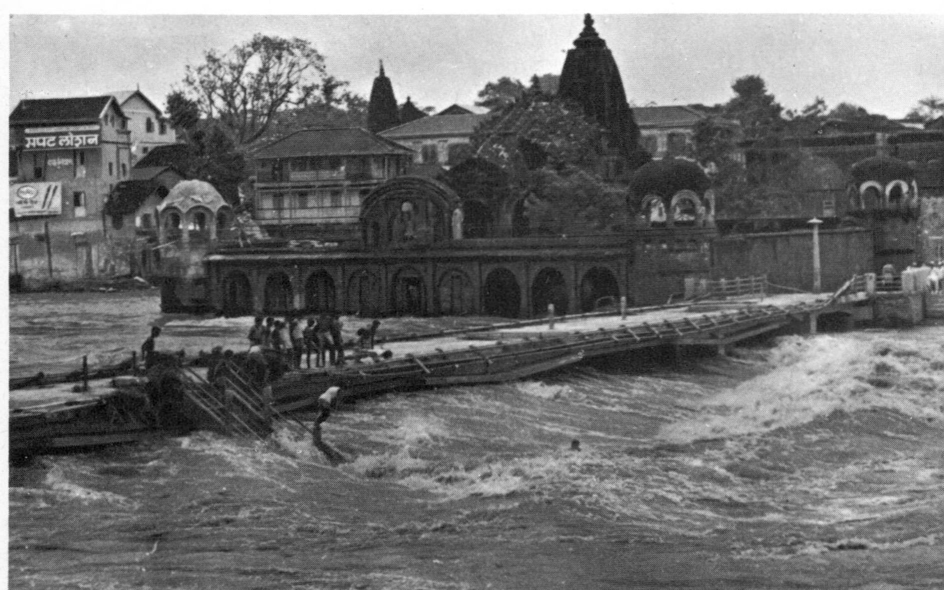

be prevented from development that will benefit the society?

Desalinated water has thrown light on the question of cost. In 1950, when Kuwait's first plant was installed, desalinated water cost as much as $\$1.25/m^3$. Subsequent development of the flash-distillation process (see Chapter 6) has reduced the price to about 25 cents/m^3, the waste heat of nuclear power plants being used as the energy source. It is likely that further improvements in technique will enable desalinated water to be delivered at a still lower cost. Who is to say what price is fair? Kuwait accepted a high one. Yet the United Kingdom has not yet accepted today's price as reasonable.

What are we to choose? Inadequate supplies at the price the uninformed public considers fair; or plentiful water at an economic price? In other words, is the price of water to be dictated by emotion or by reason? The sensible answer may be unpalatable, but it is clear. The public needs educating: it does not know the facts. It has the haziest ideas about water resources, supply and demand, pollution problems, engineering problems, and the related economic problems. It takes little interest until either the taps run dry or the streets are flooded. And then some influential newspapers, again through lack of information, misrepresent the situation, emphasize the wrong aspects, apportion blame for the wrong reasons—the public is none the wiser.

The International Hydrologic Decade

Before we consider the aims of the International Hydrologic Decade (IHD), we must define hydrology. A much-quoted definition states: "Hydrology is the science that treats of waters of the Earth, their occurrence, circulation, distribution, their chemical and physical properties, and their reaction with their environment, including their relation with living things. The domain of hydrology embraces the full life history of water on the Earth." (The Ad Hoc Panel on Hydrology of the Federal Council for Science and Technology, in a report "Scientific Hydrology," June 1962.)

While stating that the world has ample water for its needs, I have referred to the lack of precise knowledge as to the whereabouts and extents of reserves. If management is to take the decisions that will avert the threatening crisis in water, it must first know the facts. Expensive forward planning for the future cannot be based on guesswork, least of all when the public is to pay the bill.

It was recognition of the urgent need for world wide factual information on the one hand, and of the appalling gaps in the store of known facts on the other, that prompted a group of hydrologists and others to lobby for an international program of coordinated observation and research. To this end a resolution was placed before the Executive Board of UNESCO in November 1961. Calling attention to the importance of scientific hydrology, it recommended an international program over a 10-year period. Plans were drawn up and three years later the General Conference of UNESCO gave its approval. The International Decade commenced in January 1965.

Sixty of UNESCO's member nations decided to participate in the project. There are six main objectives:

1. To examine the store of existing information on world hydrology and to identify the principal gaps in present knowledge.
2. To standardize the techniques, instruments, and terminology used in hydrology all over the world.
3. To establish a world wide system for the comprehensive collection of hydrologic data.
4. To institute hydrologic research of world wide value.
5. To promote training in hydrologic science.
6. To organize systematic international exchange of hydrologic information.

The 10-year period decided on is longer than normal in international scientific programs of this nature, but was agreed upon in order to ensure the collection of sufficient data for worthwhile analysis. Rainfall, on which all surface and subterranean supplies of fresh water ultimately depend, is notoriously variable and unpredictable. It was realized, therefore, that conclusions drawn from any shorter period of observation might be significantly inaccurate.

Of the Decade's six main objectives, the first needs no elaboration. The international collection of hydrologic data is the basic aim of the entire program, and identification of the gaps in existing knowledge is a necessary preliminary if data collection is to be comprehensive.

Standardization, especially of the units and techniques of measurement, is clearly essential before information can be coordinated and comparisons made on an international basis. The planners of the Decade wisely agreed on the use of the metric system. In the area of data collection it was decided by UNESCO to concentrate on the measurement of surface- and ground-water. Apart from the fact that it is principally here that quantities are relevant to the preparation of water budgets, study of the water in the atmosphere and oceans had already been promoted in international programs of meteorology and oceanography.

Among the important data continuously required by hydrologists are measurements of rainfall, hours of sunshine, temperature, humidity, wind speed (these last four are all required for the calculation of evaporation), groundwater level (an indicator of gains and losses in groundwater reserves), and river flow.

To ensure that such measurements should be made over as wide and contiguous areas as possible, it was agreed not only to extend and improve existing networks of hydrologic observation stations, but to set up new networks. To assist in correlating the statistics at an international level, selected stations in each country were designated Decade Stations and charged with the compilation of an unusually comprehensive range of records.

In this sphere of measurement a further aim of the cooperating nations during the Decade is to improve the accuracy of measuring instruments and to devise more exact methods of estimating the total quantities of water circulating in the hydrologic cycle (see Chapter 2), especially by the development of sophisticated mechanical and electrical aids for rapid processing of collected information.

In the area of research, special studies have been instituted to integrate and interpret measurements of selected water basins all over the world. Some of these basins were chosen because they straddled national frontiers where coordinated information had hitherto been unobtainable; others because they represented internationally typical climatic, topographical, geological, or other conditions. For some of these studies areas were chosen where natural hydrologic conditions could easily be deliberately modified by man (for example by planting or cutting down large numbers of trees), in order to observe the effect of different kinds of land management on the local water cycle. Research has also been promoted in an attempt to define the boundaries, the geological texture, the capacities, and the general nature of known large groundwater reservoirs, in order to determine the relationships existing between intake and discharge areas, and to investigate the parameters that influence groundwater movement. In addition, research is being conducted internationally on the chemistry of surface- and groundwater, the effects of irrigation and drainage on the quality of groundwater, the detection of fresh groundwater by geophysical methods, and the role of vegetation in the hydrologic cycle.

Hydrology is a science to which meteorology, geology, soil mechanics, chemistry, and engineering all contribute; and since hydrologists and technicians with a useful knowledge of all these skills are rare, one aim of the International Hydrologic Decade is to promote appropriate education and training. Universities are being encouraged to expand their facilities in the relevant fields, and specialists are being made available where needed for the teaching of hydrologic science. Meanwhile a worldwide survey is being conducted to catalog all existing facilities for education in hydrology at university level. In addition, two specific aims of UNESCO during the Decade are the promotion of regional seminars and refresher courses on various aspects of the subject, and the production of up-to-date manuals and guides on the latest techniques.

The final objective of the Decade is, like the first, self-explanatory. Worldwide exchange of all collected information is a prerequisite for the success of any international scientific program. In hydrology, a science that cannot be contained within political boundaries, free exchange of information is essential to the achievement of all aims.

One of the incidental aims of the International Hydrologic Decade is to draw public attention to the role of water in modern life, and toward that aim this book is directed. In these pages I shall seek to explain, in nontechnical language, the problems and technology involved, and to stress the urgent need to use the collective talents of scientists and engineers. I hope to give pointers to the kind of imaginative planning and the bold decisions that administrators will have to make in order to prevent the potential crisis in water from becoming a reality.

The regular water crisis of drought—here in Pakistan—is the major single factor producing hardship and famine throughout the world. One of the aims of the International Hydrologic Decade is to bring the knowledge and experience of hydrologists to bear on the practical application of water conservation and irrigation techniques in those areas of the world most in need.

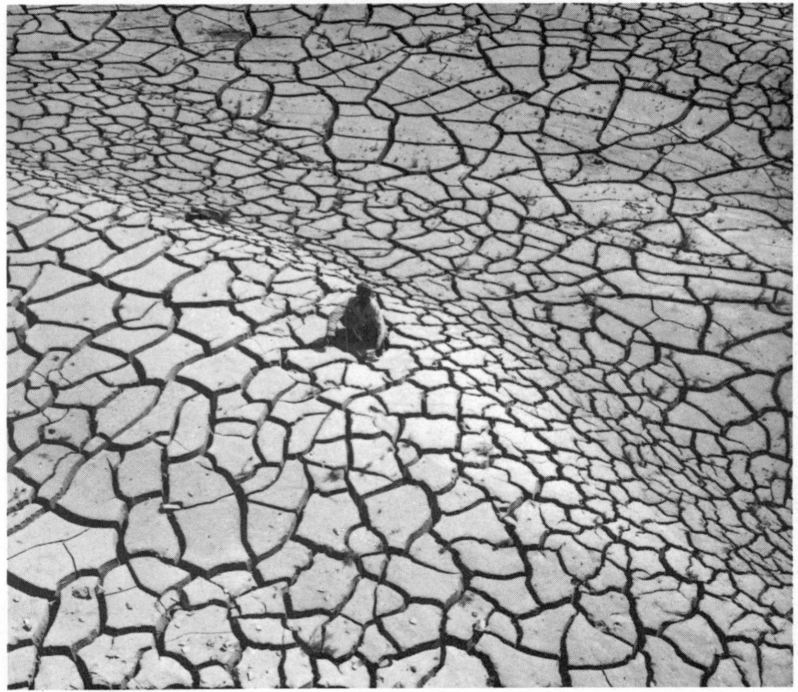

2 The Water Budget

When the sun shines hot on a sea or lake, two things happen: the surface water temperature rises, and evaporation takes place. The blanket of humid air lying over the water is itself warmed by contact with the water and, becoming lighter than the cold air above it, rises high into the atmosphere. In due course the temperature of the air falls to the point at which the water vapor begins to condense and clouds are formed. When the water droplets—or ice crystals—become too heavy to remain airborne, precipitation takes place, the water falling as rain, hail, or snow.

The Hydrologic Cycle

Much of the precipitated water falls back into the sea, but a proportion falls on land. Now four things may happen to it: (1) some water will be intercepted by vegetation and will never reach the ground; (2) some will remain on the earth's surface, dampening the soil or forming pools; (3) a proportion will seep

For centuries man has sought to modify the natural water cycle. This reservoir was built in A.D. 368 to supply Polonnaruwa, the last great capital of Ceylon.

directly into the soil; (4) the balance will form streams and begin to flow to lower ground. When precipitation stops, the water lying on vegetation and any remaining as mist in the lower atmosphere or lying in pools on the ground will begin to evaporate again. Where streams have been formed, these will flow into rivers, the water discharging eventually into lakes or the sea. And all the time a certain amount of water lying in pools or lakes, or flowing in rivers, will seep into the earth and percolate slowly down until it reaches the *water table*, the natural level of free groundwater. This water, prevented from percolating still lower by a watertight geological layer, will now tend to flow horizontally through the subsoil until it reaches land at a lower altitude, where it may reappear as a spring or artesian well, or flow from below the surface into a lake or even into the sea. Where groundwater appears above the surface, new streams are formed and the water resumes its journey overland to the sea.

But gravity is not the only force at work here. Some groundwater is drawn above the water table through the interstices (fine interconnecting spaces) in the soil by capillary action. Together with moisture percolating from above or held in the soil by molecular attraction, it may then be absorbed into the roots of vegetable matter and conveyed up into the leaves. The transpiration by the leaves returns the water, as vapor, to the atmosphere. Water that precipitates as ice or snow may remain temporarily immobile where it falls on the earth's surface. But most of this, too, will eventually reach the sea in the form of glaciers, or via rivers when it melts. Some of the melted ice and snow will seep into the ground, some will evaporate.

This whole complex process—forming a natural equilibrium of evaporation, transpiration, precipitation, surface runoff, and percolation into, and emergence from, the ground—is called the *hydrologic cycle*.

Nobody knows precisely how much water circulates in the cycle. How do we measure, and how can one visualize, water in such extravagant quantities? The commonly used metric unit of fluid measure is the liter, 1000 liters being equal to 1 cubic meter (1 m^3). Multiply a cubic meter by a million and we have 1 mega cubic meter (1 Mm^3). Multiply this by a million once again, and now we have 1 tera cubic meter (1 Tm^3). At last we have a unit of volume large enough for the measurement of the quantities of water involved in the hydrologic cycle. The following figures may be taken to represent a general consensus of expert opinion, but remember that factual data are scarce and even experts can differ.

Annual volume of water (approx.)

Evaporation		**Precipitation**	
From the sea	420 Tm^3	Over the sea	380 Tm^3
From the land	80 Tm^3	Over the land	120 Tm^3
Total	500 Tm^3	Total	500 Tm^3

At once we see that there is an estimated excess of precipitation on land totaling about 40 Tm^3, and a corresponding excess of

Water is continually moving—under the force of gravity as precipitation, runoff, and percolation, and in rising and horizontal air currents as water vapor. Storage occurs as a dynamic equilibrium of addition and depletion at four main points in the hydrologic cycle: in the atmosphere as water vapor, and in clouds as water droplets, ice crystals, and snowflakes (A); on the earth's surface in rivers and lakes and as ice and snow (B); underground in aquifers (C); and in the sea (D).

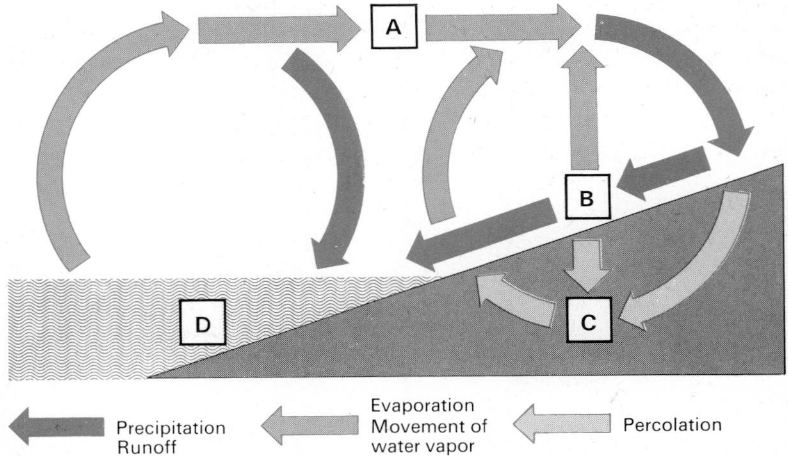

evaporation from the sea. This is the estimated quantity of water that flows annually from the land to the sea, mainly in streams and rivers.

The Energy that Drives the Cycle

The sun provides all the energy that makes the cycle work, for it is the sun's heat that evaporates the water and warms the humid air. Of the 2 million TW (a terawatt is a million million watts) of solar energy estimated to fall continuously on our planet, about 1.2 million TW reach the earth's surface, the rest being absorbed or reflected by clouds and the atmosphere. And of this 1.2 million TW, about 400,000 TW are used continuously to evaporate water. The sun's heat also raises the surface temperatures of the sea and the land, which in turn warm the lower air and cause it to rise. When precipitation takes place, some of the locked-up energy reappears. The latent heat of evaporation is released as heat, warming the air in which the

Of the total amount of solar radiation available to the earth, only a fraction, consisting of visible light and radio rays, reaches the earth's surface. Incoming infrared (heat) rays are absorbed by the atmosphere or reflected into space by clouds. However, as light rays strike the earth's surface, infrared rays are produced, and these are contained by the atmosphere. It is this reemitted heat energy that is used up in the evaporation of water.

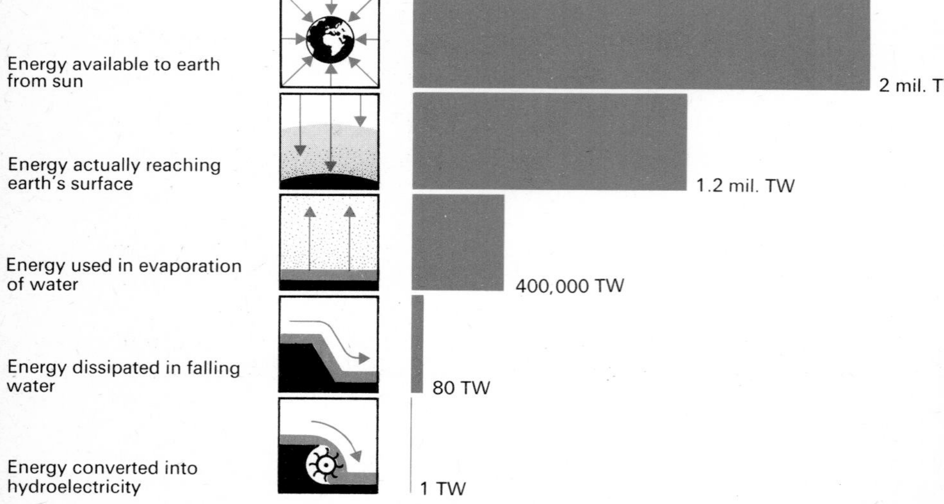

water vapor was dispersed. Some of the heat energy that warmed the vapor-laden air, causing it to rise, must clearly remain captive where rain falls at an altitude higher than that from which it evaporated. This potential energy is measured as a function of the mass of the water and its height above sea level. It is this remaining potential energy that is dissipated, mainly again as heat at an average worldwide rate of about 80 TW, as the water flows down from high ground to the sea; and it is a small part of this energy output, currently totaling about 1 TW, that the engineer converts into electrical energy in hydroelectric power plants.

Apart from its appearance in the form of rain, hail, and snow, water plays a significant part in maintaining the balance of the world's weather. If there were no water vapor in our atmosphere, not only could the significant temperature differences that cause worldwide pressure differences (and hence winds) not exist, but the absence of a heat-absorbing medium in the atmosphere would result in so great a heat loss into space that the earth's mean temperature would drop from its present average of about 15°C to approximately 0°C. Life as we know it would not exist.

World Water Resources

We have seen that some 40 Tm^3 of fresh running water are provided annually by the action of the hydrologic cycle, mainly in the form of river water. If man could impound all this fresh water he would have more than enough for all his foreseeable needs. More than half the Nile's 83,000-Mm^3 annual flow ran to waste in the sea each year before the Aswan High Dam was built, in spite of the old Aswan Dam and the various other barrages below it. More than half the water of the Indus and its tributaries, despite the world's most intensive irrigation system, runs to waste even today. And all around the world there are many other great rivers—the Yangtze, the Ganges, the Amazon, the Mississippi, the Columbia, the Volga, etc.—whose waters flow largely unexploited to the sea.

In the process of conveying 40 Tm^3 of water from the land to the sea each year, the contents of the world's rivers are changed, on average, 20 times. Thus the average capacity of all these rivers, at a given moment in time, is around 2 Tm^3. The atmosphere, through which must pass the entire 500 Tm^3 of water that circulate in the hydrologic cycle, naturally carries much more. At a given moment there are, on average, between 16 and 17 Tm^3 of water in the air—partly in the form of vapor, partly as cloud—this water precipitating and being replaced by evapotranspiration (i.e. plant transpiration plus all other evaporation) about 30 times a year. What this means may be better appreciated when we consider that the atmosphere often carries several thousand metric tons of water above a single square kilometer of the earth's surface. I mentioned in Chapter I that about 5000 Tm^3 of water (some brackish, much potable) exist within the top three-quarter kilometer of the earth's crust. True, we cannot get at all of it, and indeed may never be able to extract more than a small proportion; but consider the quantity! It is equal to the total of all the rain that would fall over the entire world's land surface in 40 years. While dealing with underground water it is of interest to mention a recent theory suggesting that water is being formed in the liquid core of the earth, the magma. Such *juvenile water*, as it is called, is thought to result either from the direct combination of hydrogen and oxygen gas, or as an expulsion from the magma or associated rocks. This theoretical underground store, were it shown to exist, would undoubtedly be the most inaccessible of all possible water sources.

To all this fresh running and underground water must be added two other reserves. One is water in the form of ice and snow, of which very considerable quantities exist at the North and South poles and on the world's many high mountain ranges. The second is the substantial store of potable water in the world's many freshwater lakes. Whether there exists any reliable estimate of the total quantity contained in the world's lakes I am unable to say: a precise estimate does exist, however, for the five Great Lakes of North America (Superior, Huron, Michigan, Erie, and Ontario), whose total capacity is approximately 22 Tm^3, half the world's annual river flow.

The capacity of the largest man-made lakes, too, is by no

means small in terms of world water reserves. Lake Kariba holds 185,000 Mm^3, Lake Nasser (Aswan) 160,000 Mm^3. Lake Bratsk and Lake Volgograd, both in the USSR, hold 179,000 Mm^3 and 32,000 Mm^3 respectively.

So much for fresh water. But if man ever found he had collected or extracted all he could reasonably reach and still wanted more, there would always be the sea from which the salts could be removed. As we shall see in Chapter 6, desalination is already used to supply fresh water in such places as Israel, Kuwait, and the southwestern states of America. As for the quantity of water in the oceans of the world, the mind boggles at the order of the figures involved. An estimate described as accurate would be suspect, but 1.6 million Tm^3 is the kind of statistic that an expert might suggest—that is, the quantity of rain that would fall on the world's land areas in well over 10,000 years. But why consider the sea as a supply of water until we have exploited the existing fresh water? And since it is the groundwater that provides the world's major reserves, let us take a closer look at it.

The Geology of Groundwater

Imagine a glass jar filled with dry coarse sand, into which some water is poured from above. What happens? The water seeps down through the fine gaps between the sand particles, displacing air, until it finds its level. Now we have a lower layer of sand that is saturated with water and an upper layer of damp but unsaturated sand (the *transition* zone). For the grains of sand now substitute a mixture of clay, sand, stone, and humus (a typical soil), or a pervious rock such as sandstone or porous limestone, and you have a picture of a water-bearing stratum, or *aquifer*, on a small scale. The bottom of the jar represents impervious underground rock, and the water level within the material in it represents the water table.

In practice an aquifer may consist of a comparatively small volume of water-filled soil or pervious rock, the water being held, as though it were an underground lake, by a depression in the lower impermeable rock. Such an aquifer may extend for a few square kilometers or less. Or it may comprise a deep layer of water-bearing strata stretching for hundreds of kilometers over a relatively level impervious rock or clay layer. An aquifer in North Africa is known to extend over an area exceeding 300,000 km^2, stretching from the middle of the Sahara Desert in the south, to the borders of Libya in the east, and to the Atlas Mountains, south of the city of Oran, in the west.

An aquifer held by a pocket in the rock surface above the general level of the water table is known as a "perched" aquifer. An aquifer can also be "confined," implying that the water-bearing stratum is trapped between two impervious layers (the North African aquifer is confined). Whenever this happens geologists recognize what they call the *piezometric surface*. This imaginary surface is the level to which the trapped water would rise, if there were no confining rock above. In practice truly confined aquifers are rare. In the first place the impermeable rock that confines them frequently contains faults through which water can leak. And if the aquifer has any outflow, however small, the water it loses must be replaced if it is to continue to exist. The area where infiltration is sufficient

Traditional methods of drawing well water are rapidly being replaced by the use of tubewells (see page 42). Here, in Malta, tradition survives. A horse drives a bucket wheel to draw irrigation water from a nonflowing artesian well.

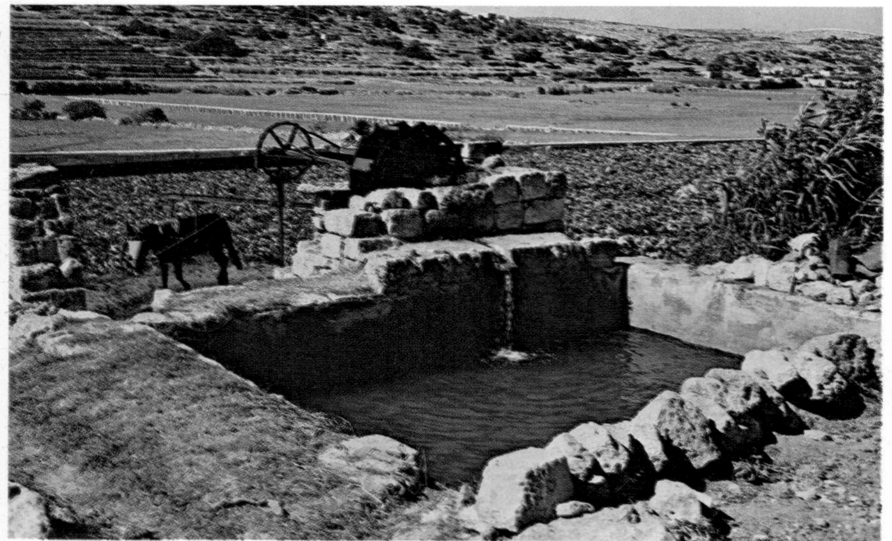

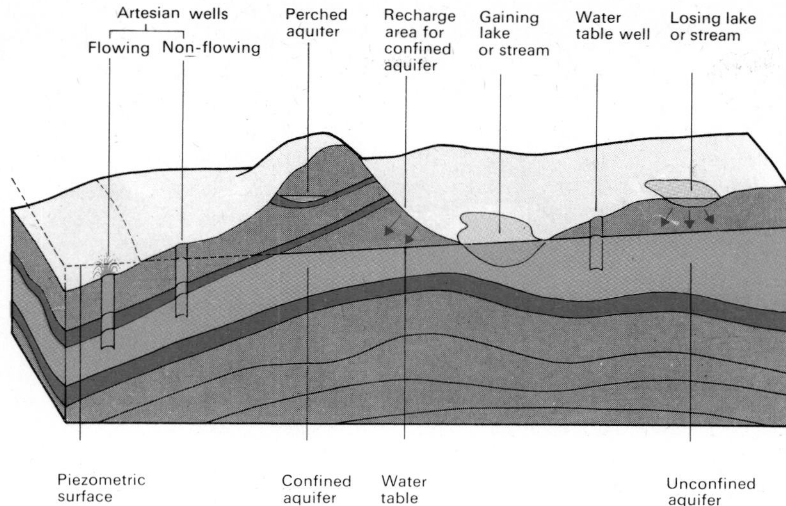

Above: hydrogeologic features shown in cross section. Impermeable rock strata (red) alternate with layers of permeable material (gray). The water table slopes from right to left. Below: when water is pumped from an aquifer, the groundwater level (A)—water table or piezometric surface—is lowered by the drawdown distance. Around a well a drawdown cone (B) is formed. Hydrologists measure the change in depth and extension of this cone, by sinking observation wells at spaced intervals from the main well, to corelate well-pumping rate with change in reserves of the aquifer. An unchanging drawdown cone indicates that the aquifer is being exploited at the safe continuous pumping rate. Where observation well measurements are unreliable, the change in depth of water in the main well is used as a criterion for determining pumping rate. Note the different route taken by groundwater when pumping from a nonflowing artesian well (left) and a water-table well (right).

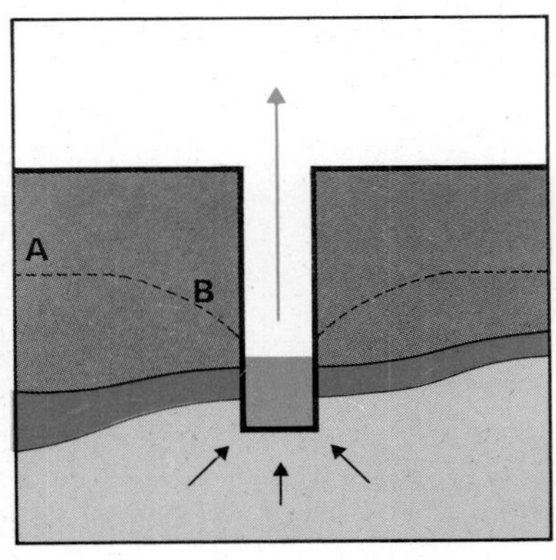

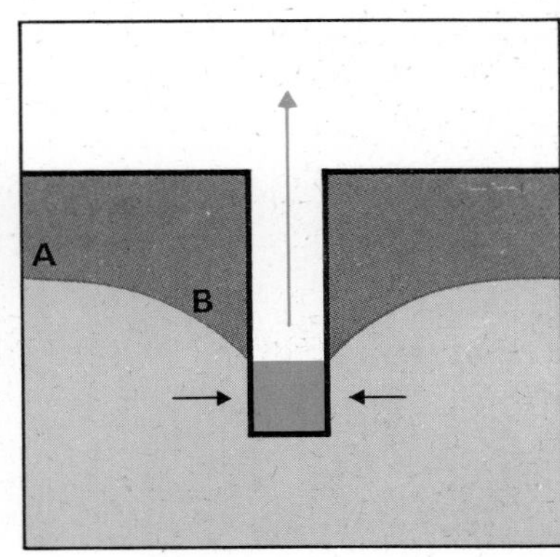

to make up for losses elsewhere is known as the *recharge area*. For confined aquifers the recharge area is usually to be found at a higher elevation, where, in fact, the aquifer is no longer confined.

When a well is dug down into an unconfined aquifer, water collects within the well at the level of the water table. If the well is pumped out, thus lowering its internal water level, the lost water is slowly replenished by groundwater infiltrating from around the well until, if pumping ceases, the original

Tubewells are used for agricultural, domestic, and industrial water supply and also for swamp reclamation. Left: water is drawn through screen filter sections of the pipe (between 20 cm. and 1 m. in diameter) by, in this case, a multistage centrifugal pump that extends into the borehole and is driven by an electric motor at the surface. A supply tubewell may be 300 m. deep and deliver water at a rate of 500 m^3/hour. Right: a tubewell being installed in West Pakistan, one of several thousand to be used in reclaiming waterlogged and saline farming land (see page 48).

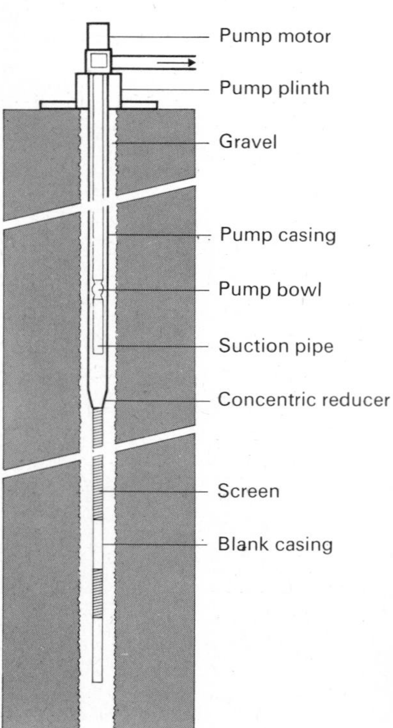

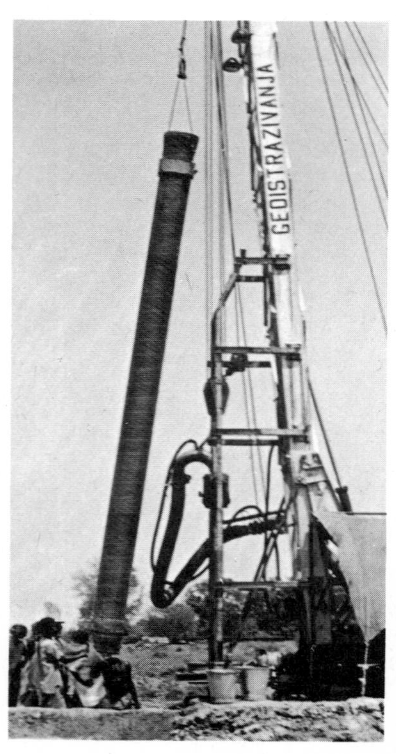

water level is again reached. When a well or borehole is drilled through rock into a confined aquifer, the water will rise to the level of the piezometric surface, and if this is above ground level (as is sometimes the case), the water will flow up and out, under pressure, as long as the aquifer continues to be replenished from elsewhere. A natural spring, where water appears from below the ground at atmospheric pressure, occurs where an unconfined aquifer breaks ground on a falling slope. Where there is a depression in the land below the water-table level, a pool or lake is formed.

Water moves underground (apart from where rock fissures or caverns have been formed) by filtering through the interstices in the soil or porous rock. This movement can take place in any direction. Rainwater or water from the bed of a stream or river percolates downward until it reaches either a layer of impermeable clay or rock, or the water table. Where it comes up against a stratum of impervious rock it will infiltrate in a generally horizontal direction, moving, as is to be expected, from higher to lower levels, until it eventually reaches the water table and becomes part of an aquifer. In other words it flows as a slow-moving underground river. This horizontal movement can vary immensely in speed, the water in slow-moving aquifers traveling as little as a few meters or less a year.

The Changing Cycle

Scientists who have observed and measured elements of the hydrologic cycle have come to the conclusion that, during the millions of years since it began to operate, it has moved steadily toward an ultimate state of dynamic equilibrium. The natural fluctuations known to occur in all the measurable variables—evaporation, transpiration, precipitation, river flow, water-table level, and some others—are merely local fluctuations, they say, that in total serve to maintain the basic trend toward equilibrium. Certainly the prime mover of the cycle, the supply of heat energy from the sun, is constant within any time scale comprehensible to man. Any observable change in the natural cycle, representing movement toward the final natural equilibrium, is caused by two basic factors: the changing nature of the earth's geography, which itself is the result of the action of water within the cycle; and biological action, upon which the water in the cycle exerts its influence.

The most obvious factor in the world's changing topography is the phenomenon of erosion. Turbulent water cuts gulleys as it passes, carrying the resulting silt in suspension to lower altitudes. There, when the water velocity drops below a certain level, the load is deposited. Glacier ice, too, erodes the rocks over which it moves. So high land is steadily cut down and low land slowly filled up. Of course the weather, itself a product of the cycle, plays a part in this erosion process. So does sand blown along by the wind.

Biological action is fostered by the results of erosion. Because lakes tend to grow shallower, century by century, as a result of the deposition of chemically rich silt on their beds, their originally pure water acquires life nutrients; microscopic organisms begin to thrive and multiply, forming in turn a biological silt on which vegetation thrives. Evidence suggests that changes of this kind occurred during prehistoric times. Variations in climate are thought to have been responsible for lakes becoming shallower and for their conversion to marshes, thereby inducing the invasion of the land by formerly completely aquatic animals. Associated hydrologic changes would be lowering of evaporation from lakes and a reduction in percolation.

I mentioned earlier that the movement of groundwater can be exceptionally slow. A method of estimating the rate of movement of a virtually stationary aquifer is by means of carbon 14 studies. One such investigation has shown that water obtained from some aquifers in the western United States has been underground some 10,000 years. If groundwater can remain interned for such long periods, the concept of a final hydrologic equilibrium loses coherence, since the very climate may change significantly before one cycle of flow in such an aquifer is complete. The historical fact of the last great ice age is a pointer here; in such circumstances one wonders how many millenniums must elapse before an equilibrium can be established!

In describing this general process of change toward a possible ultimate equilibrium I used the word "natural." This adjective is highly significant here, for there is a third factor causing change in the hydrologic cycle—the interference by man in water's natural course. And whereas the changes I have so far described are so slow as hardly to affect man within his life span, the changes he himself causes by his actions can be so rapid that they become a danger to his own continued existence if he carries them out unplanned.

Man's Interference with the Natural Cycle

Most significant of all the effects of man's interference with the hydrologic cycle is an increase in natural evaporation. By building dams he forms huge artificial lakes from the surface of which considerable evaporation takes place—as much as 25 per cent of the water thus impounded can be lost in a hot dry climate. Evaporation is increased, too, by the indiscriminate felling of forests; and the water thus gained by the atmosphere is lost elsewhere, perhaps reducing the water percolating into an aquifer that supplies a city. Or it may mean that less water flows in some local river. By pumping out groundwater and using it for irrigation agriculture, man causes above-normal evaporation from the land surface due to the soil's greatly increased moisture content. Irrigation agriculture also increases the natural transpiration rate, because it involves the replacement of natural vegetation by crops that need to transpire greatly increased quantities of water.

Man may not yet be able to alter the total of natural precipitation, but he can change its pattern by inducing rainfall where it would not normally occur; and this is a subject where researchers are at work seeking new and more efficient methods of modifying rainfall incidence for man's advantage. The pattern of natural percolation and the consequent natural recharge of aquifers is modified by several of man's activities. Dams concentrate water, causing increased percolation in the region of the huge new reservoirs. Irrigation, by spreading quantities of water on land that is normally comparatively dry, has a similar effect. The natural reappearance of groundwater is sometimes significantly augmented by pumping from tube-wells (i.e. wells of a relatively small bore lined by a pipe).

Man's interference with natural surface runoff is perhaps the most obvious of the ways in which he modifies the hydrologic cycle. Before the first Aswan Dam was built, much of the Nile's annual flow went to the sea and, by evaporation, into the atmosphere. Engineering has not reduced evaporation loss, and may have increased it, but the Aswan High Dam will eventually divert as much as 80 per cent of the water from its former destination, the Mediterranean, to the Egyptian farmers' fields. This suggests the substantial degree of interference for which man is responsible in river diversions all over the world. The desalination of seawater is, as we shall see in a later chapter, one of man's newest methods of supplying himself with fresh water. When this process becomes cheap enough to compete with other traditional methods of supply, large-scale desalination will, in effect, provide a new link in the natural cycle—a total *reversal* of natural runoff. And though much of the fresh water thus produced will doubtless find its way back into the sea after use, it will also provide a measure of aquifer recharge, the part that is not transpired or evaporated percolating into the ground, because desalinated water will probably be used in considerable quantity for agriculture.

One of the problems of water-supply engineering is that there is a wide seasonal variation in the flow of most rivers, whereas man's requirements are usually constant. Engineers therefore strive to control river flow so that the excess water of the wetter season will be available when the river would normally run low. This form of interference with the natural course of events is often achieved by means of a conventional storage reservoir from which the supply is piped direct. But sites for such reservoirs are sometimes so far from the main points of consumption that water pipes or channels to carry the water from the reservoir would be uneconomic to build and maintain. The alternative is a system of control by means of regulating reservoirs. These serve to hold up part of the river flow during the wet season, the water being released back into the river when precipitation is low. By this measure the maximum rate of extraction of water by supply undertakings downstream (a rate dictated by the minimum dry-season flow) can be significantly increased, and the river itself serves as a natural aqueduct. The United Kingdom's first reservoir of this type was opened in 1965 on a tributary of the River Dee in North Wales. By the simple expedient of building an earthfill embankment dam (see Chapter 4) and a drawoff tower containing a series of siphon tubes at different heights, engineers can control water in the river so effectively that the city of Liverpool, as a result, can take from it an additional 300,000 m^3 of water daily, this being the effective increase in the minimum dry-season flow.

One of the major (as yet unfulfilled) water schemes is the Soviet project to dam the great Ob River, which now flows northward, and divert its waters, by a system of canals, into the Aral and Caspian seas. Millions of cubic meters of fresh water now running to waste into the Arctic Ocean would thus be brought to the dry regions of western Siberia and Kazakhstan, where they could be used to irrigate many millions of hectares of currently arid land (see Chapter 8). This plan, if carried out, would constitute a highly significant major modification of the natural hydrologic cycle in the areas concerned.

The results of man's interference with the natural cycle are not always beneficial. Before the age of the dam the considerable sediments carried by the major rivers were deposited conveniently in the sea. Now, instead, the silt collects in the reservoirs formed behind the dams. Already the Hoover Dam reservoir (USA) has lost half its original capacity to waterborne sediments. The day will come when the dam will no longer serve to store water at all. In Egypt the rich silt carried down by the annual Nile flood has been used, traditionally, to fertilize the cotton fields; the natural deposit on one hectare (2.471 acres), at today's prices, is equivalent to $10-worth of man-made fertilizer. Today, though Egypt has more water for her agriculture than ever before, the Nile no longer carries the fertile sediments of upland erosion into the fields it waters; instead the silt is now trapped by the new Aswan High Dam (the old dam was designed to let much of the floodwater through—silt and all). To offset this loss the High Dam project incorporates a huge hydroelectric generation plant that will be used to power an enormous fertilizer factory as well as to supply electricity for other domestic and industrial needs.

Another disturbing consequence of man's interference with the natural cycle is the ruination of hundreds of thousands of hectares of fertile cropland by the very act of irrigation. Natural water, especially groundwater, contains a small proportion of dissolved mineral salts. Since the whole system of irrigation in hot, dry areas results in very considerable evaporation, the salt content of the unevaporated water increases slowly but steadily, until the concentration of salts in the transition zone from which the crops draw their water becomes higher than the crops can tolerate. There is now only one course open—that of attempting to leach out the accumulated salts by additional irrigation designed to cause percolation of the salts, in solution, deeper down into the ground.

Misuse of the soil and interruption of the natural hydrologic cycle can result in uncontrolled soil erosion and loss of fertility. Here, in Georgia, USA, good land goes to waste after many years of farming mismanagement.

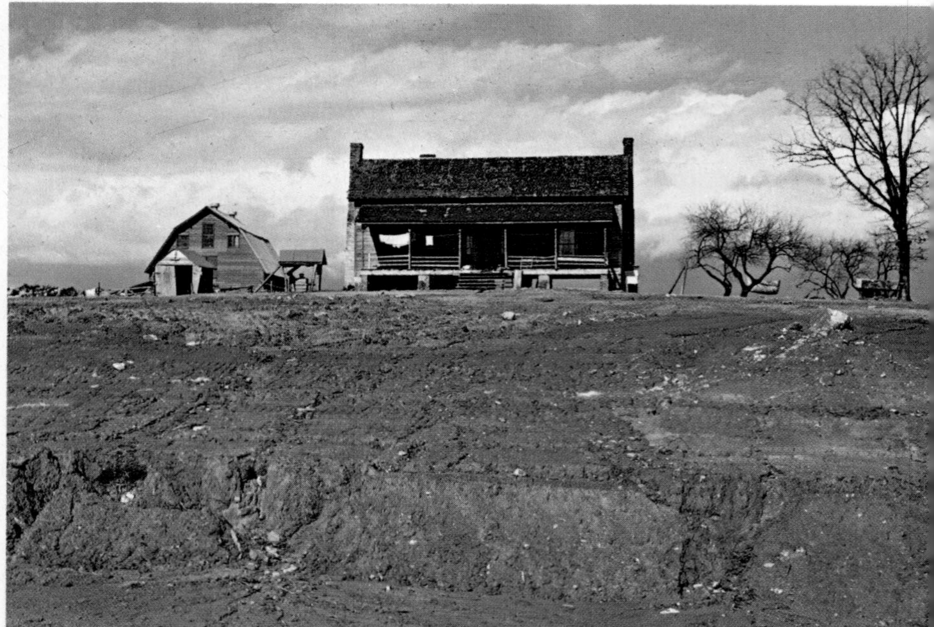

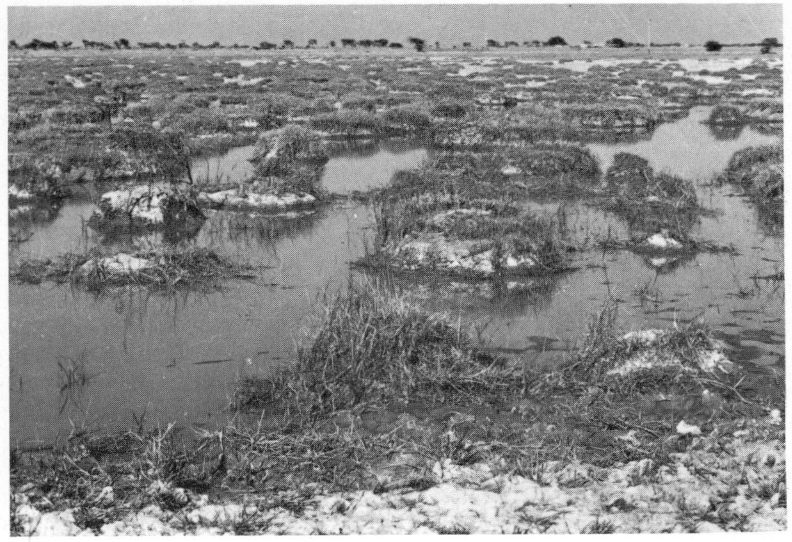

Above: the effects of over-irrigation in West Pakistan. Rapid evaporation from the soil surface has resulted in an increase in the salt content of water in the root zone to a level above that tolerated by the crops. Attempts to leach out accumulated salt by further irrigation have raised the water table and produced waterlogging. Below: hydrologists at the West Pakistan Irrigation Research Institute, Mandipur, are using model layouts in order to develop more efficient irrigation techniques.

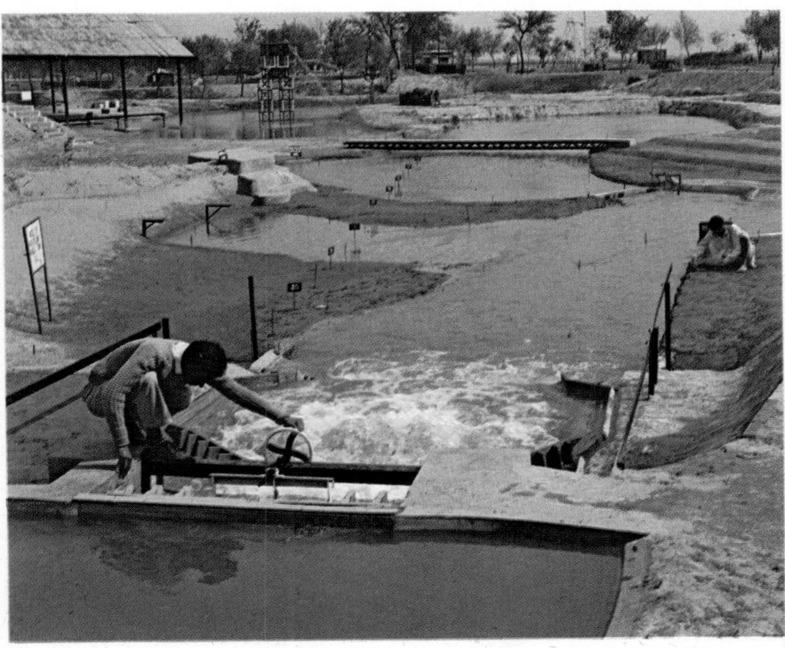

Unfortunately, as heavy irrigation serves to raise the water-table level, this practice often results in the land becoming waterlogged. The plant roots have no access to air and the crops fail due to lack of oxygen. So serious has this problem of soil salinity become in West Pakistan, vast areas of which are irrigated by river barrages and associated canal systems, that 40,000 hectares of valuable food-producing land are currently being lost to cultivation each year. Where such land has been abandoned and irrigation stopped, the salt can be seen lying thick and white on the ground. What was once a desert, before the engineer came and rendered it richly fertile by irrigation, has once again become a desert due to man's interference with the natural water cycle.

A further undesirable consequence of irrigation works is that of erosion equilibrium with time, the channel enlarging itself until it is big enough to carry the normal flow without further erosion of its banks. By building dams man creates a situation in which large volumes of water must lose height very rapidly. If the channels for this water are not to be eroded they must be lined with materials such as concrete. Thus in areas of scenic beauty an aesthetic problem is created. Concrete banks also make flood control more of a problem, because they cannot absorb water temporarily as the porous banks of natural watercourses do in areas prone to flooding.

Excessive groundwater pumping can have unsatisfactory consequences apart from the growing salinity caused by increased evaporation. The water table will probably be lowered (in a confined aquifer the hydrostatic pressure will drop), and rivers and springs lose instead of gain water, sometimes drying up as a result. One consequence of groundwater development may thus be the reduction in potential hydroelectric power output of the area—an unfortunate result, because the very act of pumping groundwater requires power. So the engineer may well find himself robbing Peter to pay Paul. Excessive pumping from a confined aquifer may also cause elastic deformation of the water-bearing strata. Lowering the water table by pumping from unconfined aquifers sometimes increases the hydraulic gradient so significantly that the aquifer will yield more water than in its natural state; on the other hand the resulting increase in the pumping "head" may make the whole operation uneconomic in terms of the cost of water produced.

Even the building of cities affects the hydrologic cycle, sometimes to man's loss, since extensive paving and other coverage of the ground surface from the rain may, in fact, deprive an aquifer of its recharge area. If the aquifer feeds the city's water-supply system the growth of the city tends to reduce the water available to it.

What the advantages and disadvantages of man's interference with the hydrologic cycle will finally add up to is not easy to foretell. Certainly the uneasy state of natural equilibrium becomes more unstable, and even more unpredictable. We cannot, therefore, hope to forecast with any certainty how traditional sources of water will react to man's action; and with the water demand growing so rapidly, those who must make vital decisions are left in a dilemma.

Before we can go further into the question, however, we must know how the hydrologist attempts to measure the various elements in the cycle. Accurate measurement of current water movement and the scientific evaluation of trends is the planner's only hope.

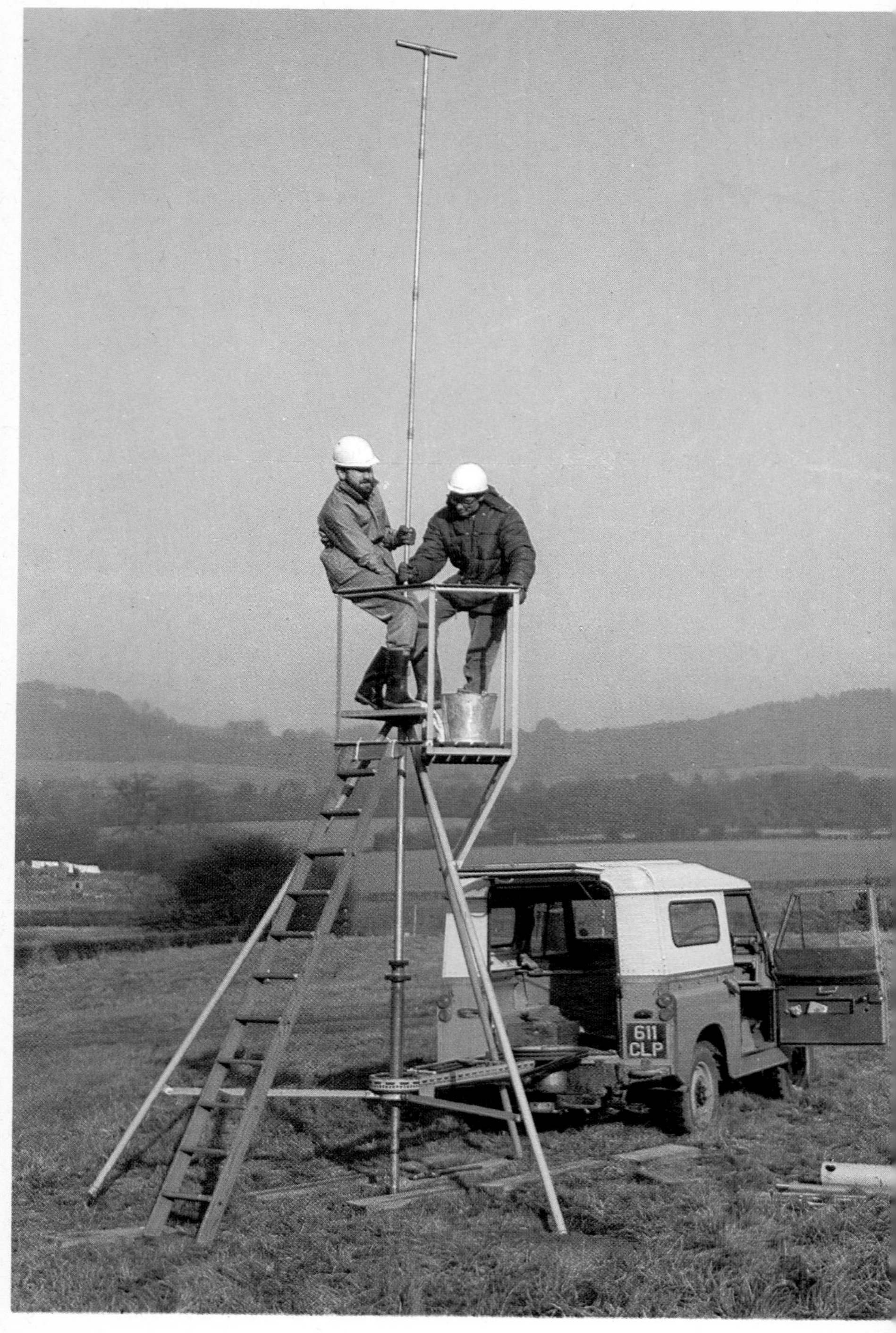
611
CLP

3 Measuring Water

It is all too easy to talk glibly of the vast quantities of water that circulate in the hydrologic cycle but actually measuring them is not so easy. You cannot fit a flow meter to a river. Nor can you catch and measure the rain that falls, shall we say, in a 10-minute cloudburst over the Alps, or check the volume of an artesian aquifer that may be 10 km. long. You cannot weigh a cloud.

If the world's water resources are to be budgeted and properly exploited, we must have accurate estimates, if not always measurements, of the quantities of water involved. How then does the hydrologist measure the enormous quantities of water that circulate in the hydrologic cycle? He can measure the water velocity at any particular point in a river, but this may vary widely from bank to bank, and from river bed to surface. The water may cascade over rapids, and hardly seem to move in a deep, wide reach below. Even if a relationship can be established between the water velocity at a particular point and the total

Hydrologists sinking a stainless steel access tube in preparation for neutronic ground-moisture measurement (see page 59).

flow, this is likely to vary significantly if the water level rises or falls, as it is bound to do in response to the variations in rainfall that may occur anywhere within the catchment area. Similar difficulties arise in the compilation of other hydrologic data. We can measure rainfall at a given location over a given period. But this measurement does not necessarily reflect the total rainfall in any particular area around that location. There might have been a local downpour.

Even greater problems arise when one thinks in terms of measuring evaporation and transpiration rates. Evaporation can only be measured simply when it takes place from a free water surface; so evaporation from the ground or from vegetation must be computed from measured water surface evaporation by using coefficients that will vary from one situation to another. Nor do measurements and calculations for any one location necessarily bear a fixed relationship to the evaporation and transpiration that will take place at another, however near.

In any case, any measurement we may make of evapotranspiration is necessarily indirect; one can in no way trap the water vapor loss from a field of wheat or rice or potatoes, or from plowed land or grazing, over a given period of time, and weigh or otherwise measure it. Moreover, the actual evapotranspiration rate can vary significantly from minute to minute in response to changes in humidity, temperature, sunshine, wind speed, and rainfall.

When he comes to the measurement of groundwater the hydrologist must face yet another difficulty: he cannot see the water, nor sometimes does he know its precise location. Even spot readings, however accurate and however widely located, may be of little value on their own. For though the hydrologic cycle, as we have seen, is a process moving constantly toward a total equilibrium, specific water movement within its many facets is a changing phenomenon; it changes hourly, daily, seasonally, and annually. For the hydrologist to be able to draw up a picture general enough in scope and sufficiently accurate in detail to be of real value to him and to the engineer, he must not only have correct readings distributed widely in terms of space, but must have continuous data collected over long periods of time covering all normal seasonal weather variations. The collected measurements are analyzed and assembled in the form of continuous hydrologic "maps." Until comparatively recent times these maps were hopelessly incomplete. However diligently a country with a water problem might have sought and assembled the required information, a neighboring country might have done little or nothing, leaving water movement across the borders a totally unknown quantity. Yet such movement might be highly significant to the less favored country's water budget. Fortunately the International Hydrologic Decade is playing an important role in solving this problem and today, for the first time, it has become possible to compile relatively comprehensive hydrologic maps as a result of the worldwide collection, standardization, and exchange of information.

The Hydrologic Equation

Fortunately for the hydrologist, there is a basic equation, a comparatively simple manifestation of the law of conservation of matter, that aids him in finding his way through the maze of hydrologic data. This equation, in its simplest form, is:

Total inflow = Total outflow + Total change in storage.

In nature, fortunately, water remains water; it does not change chemically. So in a given period of time the total flow of water into a defined area must equal the outflow plus the change in storage. Devastatingly obvious though the equation might appear, it dominates the field of hydrologic measurement for the simple reason that every unknown is concerned with one of the three functions; so every measurement can be checked or, where a particular measurement cannot be made with any degree of accuracy, it can be calculated from others. It must be remembered, of course, that the validity of the equation depends on the word "total" in its definition. To compute total inflow we must know precipitation, surface inflow, groundwater inflow, and artificial import (such as water piped or channeled in). Similarly total outflow must include evaporation, transpiration, surface outflow, artificial export, and *interception loss* (precipitation intercepted by foliage, buildings, etc., and returned to the atmosphere by evaporation without having ever reached the ground). Total change in storage must include variations in the quantity of stored groundwater, of soil moisture (that is, water in the transition zone), of water standing in lakes and reservoirs, and of channel storage (defined as water actually flowing, and hence temporarily stored while in motion) in rivers and other water channels.

The contemporary hydrologist has a wide array of instruments and equipment to help him in his task. The most crude, but still probably the most widely used, is the nonrecording rain gauge, in which rain is caught by a large circular funnel, led into a narrow cylindrical tank, and measured at intervals with a measuring jar or a calibrated dipstick. Among the most sophisticated of his tools is the analogue computer, designed to measure the movement of underground water in every direction in a given area. Such a computer (described later in this chapter) can quickly provide information vital to the engineer in an area in which large-scale tubewell pumping is planned or is being carried out. Between these two extremes lies a wide range of current meters, water-level recorders, evaporation pans, *lysimeters* (to measure the rate of vertical infiltration of water into soil), snow-surveying equipment, and numerous other items.

Measurement of Precipitation

While the simple rain gauge is still widely used, the recording rain gauge, which provides continuous information, is superseding it. Early models, operated by clockwork, made a graph of the weight of the water collected by the gauge. Today electric actions replace the clockwork, and electronics either records the information on punched paper or magnetic tape or conveys it direct to the nearest hydrologic station. A comparatively recent development in rain-reading techniques is the use of radar for estimating the precise area affected by storm showers. Readings from rain gauges within the storm area are used in conjunction with the radar information to obtain a far more accurate estimate of storm precipitation than had been possible by earlier methods. The effect of wind has always been a problem and no means has yet been found to prevent it affecting the accuracy of a rain gauge's "catch." So this, along with errors caused by the location of a gauge (on a tall building, perhaps, where a suitable open space does not exist) are taken care of by the use of mathematical formulas evolved over the years as a result of painstaking research.

Rain, of course, is not the only form of precipitation. Snowfall, too, has to be measured. One difficulty in measuring snowfall accurately is the fact that a percentage of it often melts after it has fallen but before a measurement has been made. To compensate for this error the hydrologist employs a series of equations relating snowmelt to the various possible causes (air convection, vapor condensation, radiation, precipitation of warm rain, conduction from the earth, and conduction from the air). In practice, where snowfall and runoff records have been kept over several years, it is often possible to establish a relationship between the two. In this way snowfall measurement can be used to forecast spring and summer runoff without the

Radar pictures of a heavy rainstorm. Left: as recorded by the circular sweep of a plan position indicator radar (PPI). Right: as recorded by a range height indicator (RHI). Distances are in miles and height is in thousands of feet.

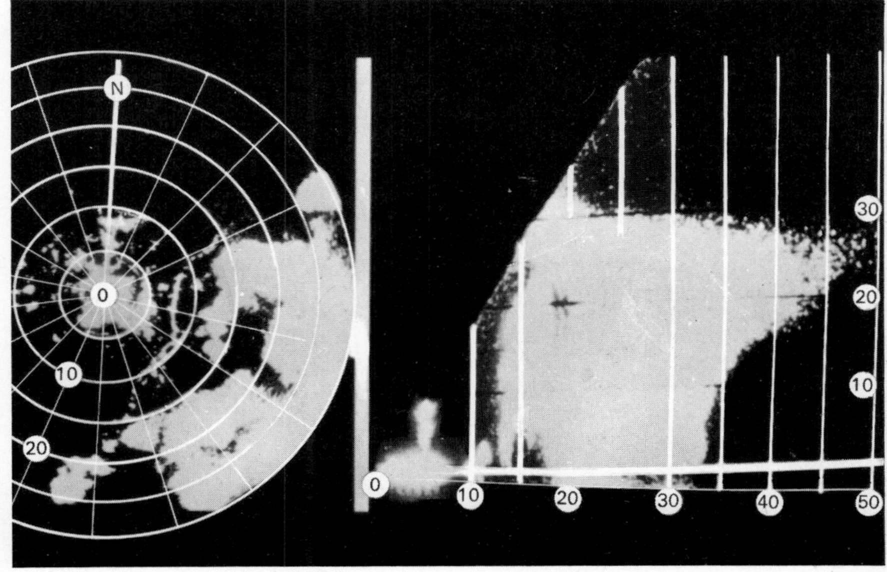

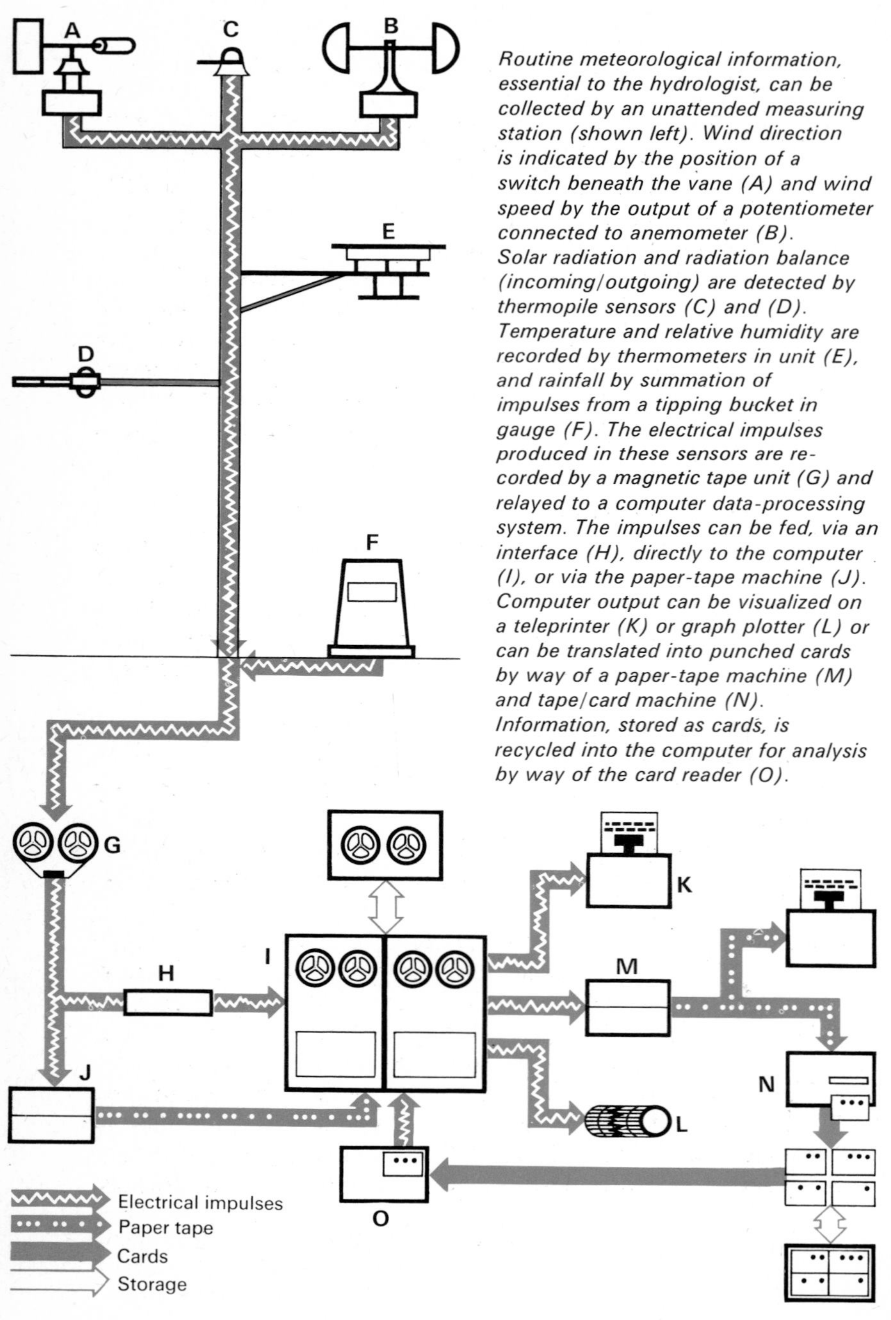

Routine meteorological information, essential to the hydrologist, can be collected by an unattended measuring station (shown left). Wind direction is indicated by the position of a switch beneath the vane (A) and wind speed by the output of a potentiometer connected to anemometer (B). Solar radiation and radiation balance (incoming/outgoing) are detected by thermopile sensors (C) and (D). Temperature and relative humidity are recorded by thermometers in unit (E), and rainfall by summation of impulses from a tipping bucket in gauge (F). The electrical impulses produced in these sensors are recorded by a magnetic tape unit (G) and relayed to a computer data-processing system. The impulses can be fed, via an interface (H), directly to the computer (I), or via the paper-tape machine (J). Computer output can be visualized on a teleprinter (K) or graph plotter (L) or can be translated into punched cards by way of a paper-tape machine (M) and tape/card machine (N). Information, stored as cards, is recycled into the computer for analysis by way of the card reader (O).

laborious task of computing the likely snowmelt from these various causes.

Once regular readings of precipitation are available at specific locations in an area, there follows the problem of analyzing the data and building up a precipitation map covering the entire area. That such analysis is not easy will be clear when one stops to think how variable rainfall can be even in the long term, and how rapid the variations can be in the short. Also there is the problem that precipitation data are often required for areas that do not coincide with the locations of established rain gauge stations. Fortunately the hydrologist has an ally here in the relationships that have been found to exist between precipitation and geography, though the equations are numerous and sometimes complex.

Groundwater Measurement

There are four measurements that the hydrologist needs to make of groundwater. These are (1) the volume of an aquifer, for which he must know both the effective area and the mean thickness; (2) the elevation of the water table or piezometric surface; (3) the speed of groundwater movement; and (4) the specific yield of the aquifer.

To detect the presence of an aquifer, borehole samples are taken and examined in order to identify the various strata present. This is followed by one or more of the following techniques:

(1) Resistivity testing, which is based on the fact that water-bearing strata conduct electricity more readily than similar strata that are dry.

(2) Seismic refraction analysis, using shock waves, the results of which can give positive indications of the presence of water.

(3) Measurement of neutron or gamma ray absorption parallel with the wall of a well, a technique (sometimes known as "well logging") that can supply valuable information on the structure and water content of the aquifer through which the well passes.

Measurement of the elevation of the water table depends on the existence of a well or borehole. Recording float gauges are widely used, but a simple technique requiring only a small bore tube from ground level to the water uses air pressure to calculate the depth of the water table (see page 62).

The speed at which groundwater flows can in theory be calculated, provided the hydraulic gradient and permeability coefficient are known. Unfortunately both may vary significantly along the course of an aquifer's flow, and calculation is usually impracticable. Direct methods of measurement have been evolved, however, involving the use of nontoxic tracers, which are introduced into the aquifer at a suitable location, their passage to some other point of access being timed. Radioactive tracers, such as tritium, deuterium, and oxygen 18, can be followed above ground by Geiger counter, thus providing a means of continuous groundwater velocity measurement over a distance. Also, as we have already seen, carbon 14 is found in some aquifers where recharge and discharge are separated by many hundreds of years. Since, like all radioactive substances, this carbon isotope disintegrates at a known fixed rate, the expert can use its concentration to calculate the time that has elapsed since the water containing it entered the aquifer at its recharge area. He can then compute its average velocity underground.

The only satisfactory method of measuring the specific yield of an aquifer (the quantity of water that can be continuously withdrawn) is by well-pumping tests. Specific yield is the

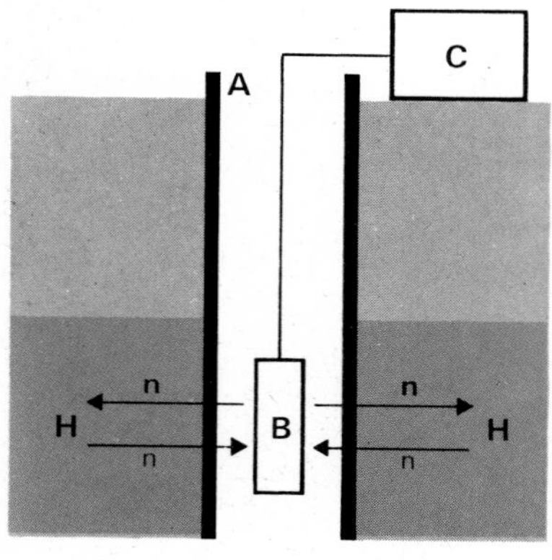

*Neutronic moisture measurement. A stainless steel tube (A) is sunk into the ground and the probe (B) inserted. Fast neutrons (**n**) are emitted, which, by collision with the hydrogen atoms (H) of water molecules, are converted to slow (thermal) neutrons (n). The probe is sensitive to the density of these low-energy particles and the number is registered on the counter (C). Count of slow neutrons per unit time provides an accurate measurement of water content.*

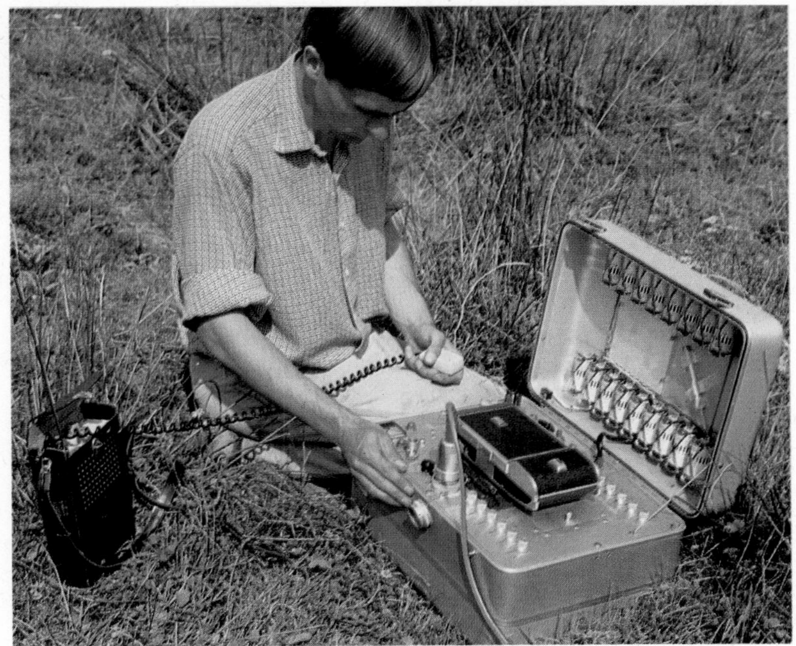

Surveying for water, using the seismic refraction technique. An explosion is set off and seismic waves are relayed by way of 12 geophones (electromechanical detectors) to a 12-channel oscillograph (above). The wave-refraction patterns, which vary according to the water content of the underlying rock, are recorded on a polaroid camera plate (below right).

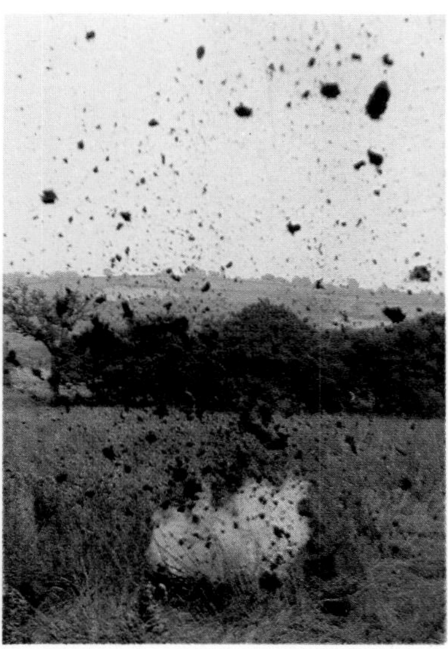

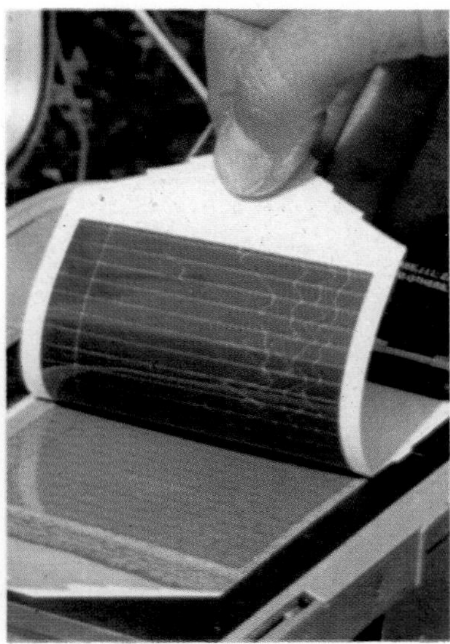

fraction of the saturated bulk volume of the aquifer consisting of water that will drain by gravity when the water table drops. It rarely exceeds 30 per cent, and can be calculated, using the hydrologic equation; however, it requires the collection of a great deal of data and is a laborious and error-prone process.

The problem of relating point measurements to water movement patterns over an area is as basic in the study of groundwater behavior as in precipitation analysis. Here, however, the electronics engineer has provided the hydrologist with a valuable new tool. Point measurements of permeability, storage coefficients, and water-table level are used to build up an electronic network representing the area under study. Resistors represent permeability, capacitors the storage capacity, voltages the pressure "head" depending on the water-table level. The

Left: an automatic water-elevation recording station. Measurements are taken over a stilling well (A) to allow for deepening of the channel. The recorder datum (B) is fixed at the lowest foreseeable water level. The vertical height above the datum of the counterweighted float (C) is registered as a line hydrograph on a revolving drum. On the inset graph the pen has reversed direction to record the peak of a flood (D). Staff gauge (E) is used for rapid visual checking. Right: air-line measurement of water-table depth. Pump (F) supplies compressed air through the gauge (G) to an air line of known length (H). The pressure recorded when all the water is blown out indicates the depth of water to the bottom of the air line (I). The distance between ground level and the water table (J) can thus be calculated.

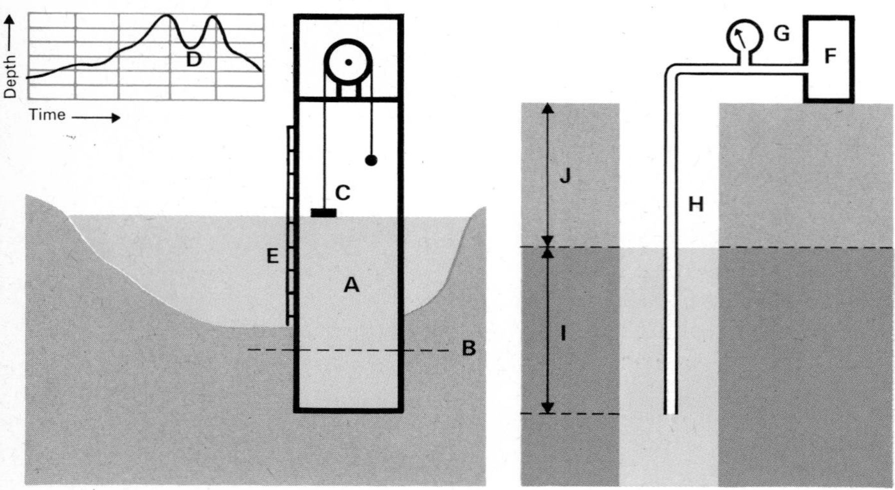

electric currents that now flow in the various links of the network simulate the water flow. Once such an analogue computer has been built up for an area the total effect of changing any of the variables in any part of the area can be quickly measured. This system is proving particularly valuable in determining the variation in groundwater level that will occur throughout a large aquifer when water is pumped out at various rates and at various locations. One such computer is the basis of the control center of London's latest groundwater supply project.

Apart from the analogue computer, physical analogue models are also sometimes used to study groundwater movement. One such, used with success in Israel, employs oil in a narrow gap between a pair of vertically placed glass plates to simulate a vertical section of water-bearing rocks. Oil dropped in from above represents freshwater replenishment, holes in the back plate providing means to draw off oil, thereby simulating the effect of pumping. Two oils of different color have even been used in the Israeli analogue model to study the underground interface between fresh groundwater and salt water infiltrating under the coast from the sea.

Measurement of Surface Runoff

Stream gauging is one of the hydrologist's most basic tasks. It not only contributes to the calculation of the total water resource, but provides minimum and maximum flow data information vital to the engineer who designs flood control works, irrigation barrages, or dams for hydroelectric projects. The oldest known example of stream gauging is to be found in the centuries-old "Nilometers," calibrated posts driven by the ancient Egyptians into the bed of the river Nile. Continuous records of the maximum flood height of the Nile, kept at the Roda (Cairo) Nilometer, are available almost without a break from A.D. 622 to 1521, and contemporary corelation studies, relating the high water level to the mean flood flow, have given the hydrologist a unique insight into the Nile's behavior over many hundreds of years.

Modern stream gauging comprises two correlated measurements: that of water-surface elevation, and that of total discharge. Measurements of infiltration into the ground, of interception loss, and of evapotranspiration are also required in order to complete the hydrologic equation linking runoff with precipitation.

As the water level in rivers often changes rapidly, staff-gauge readings on the Nilometer principle can be misleading. The maximum water level may be missed between regular readings in times of storm and cloudburst. In the low-water season the day–night temperature variation may alter the evapotranspiration rate so significantly as to result in a marked discharge cycle in small rivers, again resulting in misleading information from regularly timed staff-gauge readings. Consequently the modern recorder is an automatic instrument that records water elevation continuously against time.

The measurement of stream discharge is a more complex operation owing to the variations in water velocity that occur from bank to bank, from bed to surface, and from source to

Hydrologists collecting streamflow and meteorological data at South Cascade Glacier, Washington, USA, for the IHD. They are constructing a measuring weir at the outlet of the glacier's terminal lake. Instruments in the shelter record air temperature, wind speed, and summer precipitation.

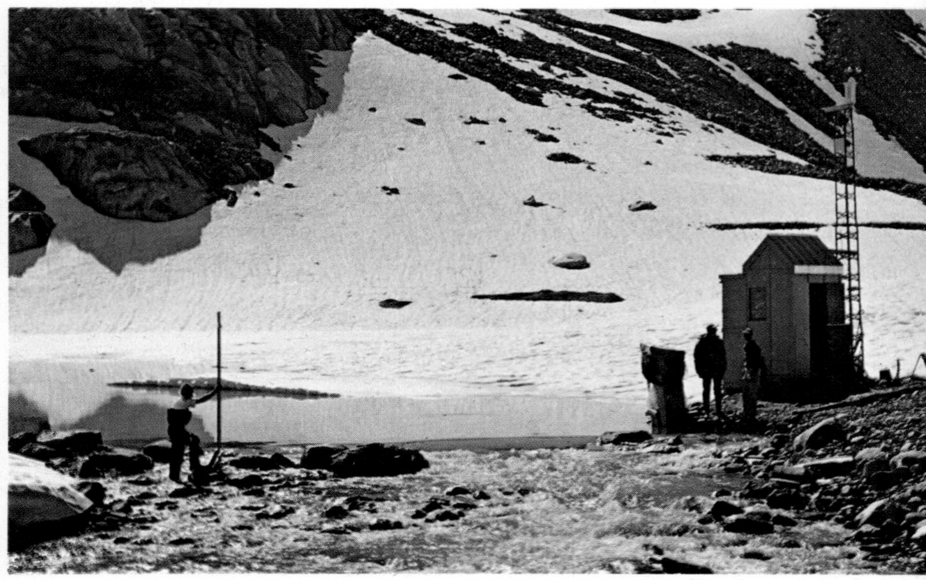

mouth of the river. These variations depend on the profile of the river bed, on the bends in the river's course, and on the resulting friction to flow. Where convenient, this problem can be solved by diverting the entire water flow through a weir incorporating a measuring device, such as a "V" notch or venturi flume. As the water passes through this restricted opening, drop in water level or lowering of hydrostatic pressure is used as a measure of flow rate. Stream diversion is, of course, not usually possible. In this case the stream is divided arbitrarily into cross-sectional areas, the water velocity in each area being measured with a current meter. The discharge within each area is then calculated and the total stream discharge computed.

Infiltration, Evaporation, and Transpiration

Hydrologists recognize a constant, known as the *infiltration* (or *f*-) *capacity* for any given sample of land. This is the maximum rate at which water can percolate into the soil surface.

Scientists using a groundwater analogue computer at the Water Research Association Centre, England, to study aquifer exploitation and recharge.

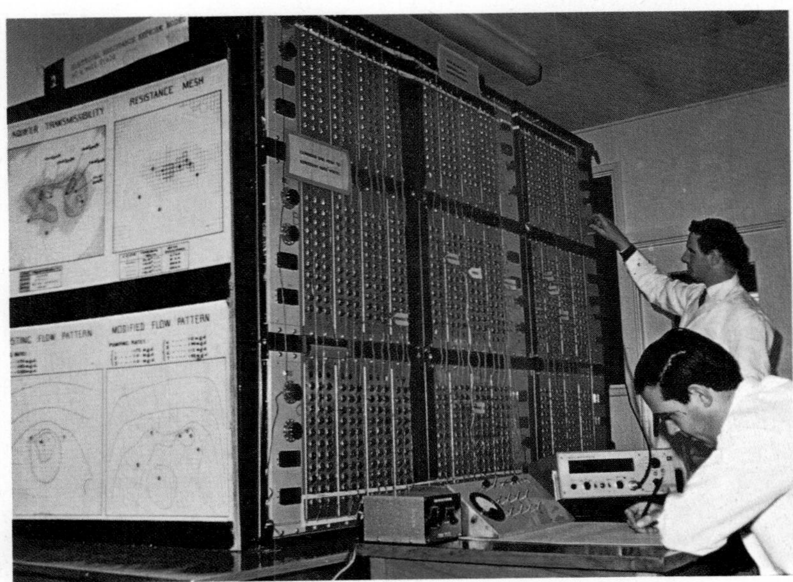

While the f-rate for a given area can, in theory, be calculated mathematically using the results of soil analysis, the hydrologist is once again faced with so many elusive variables that he prefers more direct methods of computation based on the hydrologic equation already described. Direct measurement is also possible by the application of water to an experimental plot at known rates by sprinkler, measuring the maximum that can be visibly absorbed, and the placing of a lysimeter under the land, enabling infiltrating water to be drawn off and measured.

Interception loss can be computed by measuring the water that a given sample of vegetation can hold against the action of gravity and the wind (a typical figure is 1 mm. of rainfall), and by solving an equation using the known evaporation rate in measured conditions of humidity, temperature, and wind speed. Interception loss is usually of the order of 12 per cent of total precipitation.

We have seen how very considerable quantities of precipitated water escape from the land by the combined process of evapotranspiration. Direct field measurement of evaporation and transpiration is wholly impracticable, and once again computation relies on solution of the hydrologic equation, and requires direct measurement of the basic rate of evaporation from a free water surface in the area concerned. This is achieved by means of the evaporation pan. Since direct readings have to be modified by corelation coefficients related to the relative humidity, temperature, and wind speed, an evaporation station invariably includes instruments to measure these variables, and a rain gauge so that the quantity of rain falling into the pan is also known.

While the rate of evaporation from the land depends only on temperature, humidity, and wind speed, and can easily be calculated, transpiration is also related to the type of vegetation and the quantity of plant tissue being synthesized, itself dependent on sunshine. Calculation of transpiration rates is consequently more involved. However, a constant known as the *transpiration ratio* (the weight of water required for transpiration in the production of unit weight of dry plant tissue—for common grain crops it varies between 500 and 600) can be made use of if the crop or vegetation growth in a known period can be weighed. Alternatively, experimental data providing mean transpiration rates for various types of vegetation under typical climatic conditions may be used for estimating. Wheat, for example, is known to transpire about 300 mm. of water a year in a typical temperate climate.

A primary difficulty in correlating hydrologic data on a worldwide basis has been the total lack of standardization in units of measurement, and consequently in the specifications of the special measuring instruments concerned. While a major proportion of the world's hydrologic data has traditionally been based on the British system of weights and measures, one of the tasks undertaken during the International Hydrologic Decade is to obtain agreed metric standards for the measurement and presentation of hydrologic data of all kinds. As I have already mentioned, in this book I have abandoned the traditional Western unit for the measurement of large quantities of water (the acre-foot) in favor of the simple metric cubic meter. Perhaps, by the time the Decade has ended, the physical dimensions of such instruments as the simple rain gauge will have been standardized in terms of metric units, and the substantial, but essential, task of replacing the hundreds of thousands of instruments based on the British system of weights and measures and currently in use over many parts of the world will be well in hand.

One final word on water in the balance. Measurement of the water that circulates in the hydrologic cycle is, as we have seen, vital to effective water management. Yet, despite the instruments, techniques, and formulas I have described, the hydrologist of 1968 is at a great disadvantage compared with men in probably every other scientific field. Hydrology is still, to a great extent, an art—one that Samuel Mandel, a leading Israeli hydrologist, has described as "the art of inferring the right conclusions from woefully inadequate data."

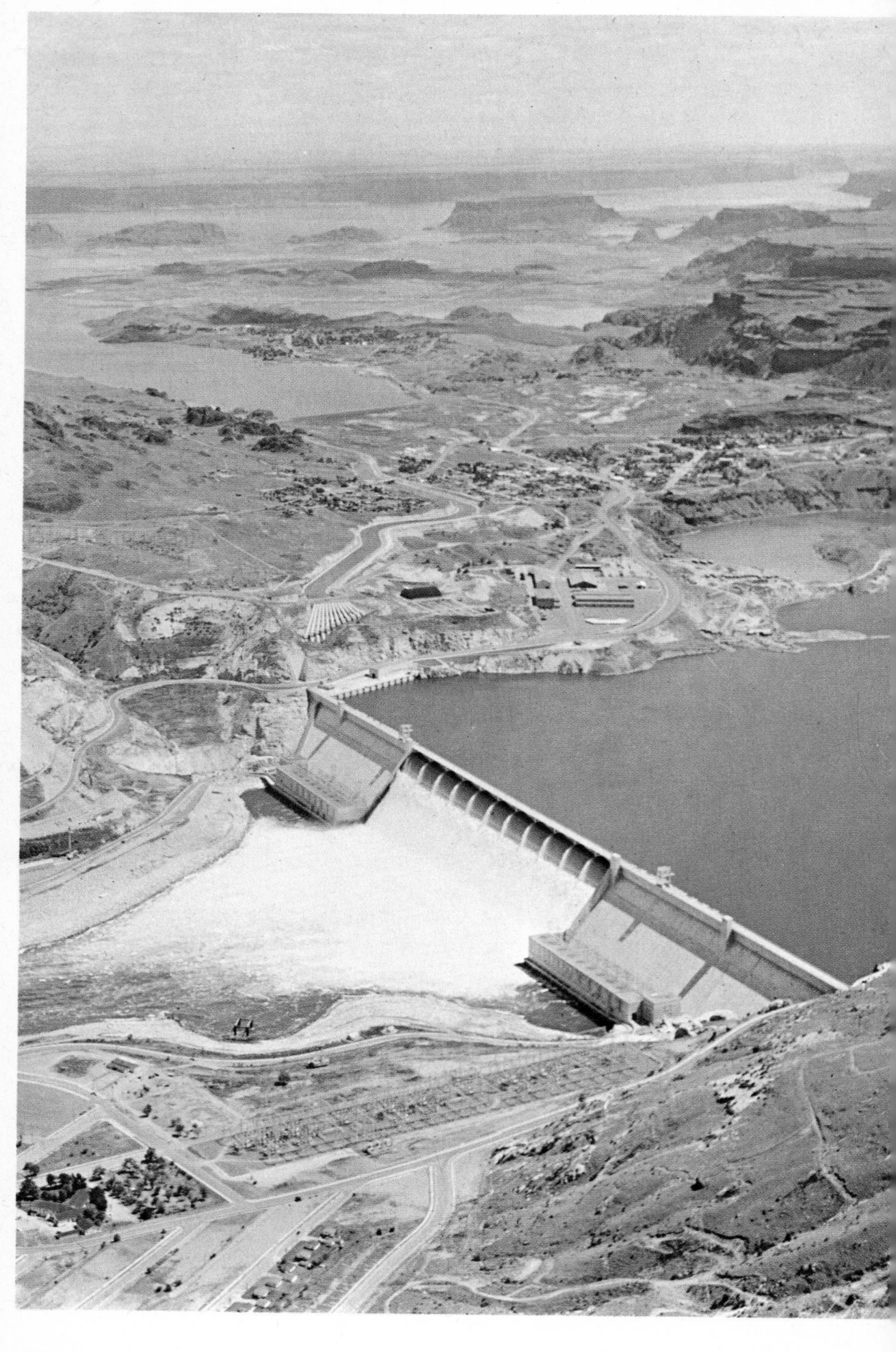

4 Irrigation and Dams

Engineering for the supply of water for irrigation and for domestic use involves three distinct technologies: the civil engineering of barrages and dams and their associated water distribution channels and tunnels; the mechanical engineering of raising water from a lower to a higher level; and the chemical engineering of water purification. The last, which today has two entirely separate facets—the removal of general impurities from polluted water, and the desalination of naturally occurring salt water—will be the subject of later chapters. In this chapter we shall look at the technologies of barrage- and dam-making, and of pumping and water distribution, and learn something of their early history.

The History of Water Engineering

It is recorded that 5000 years ago King Menes of Egypt dammed the Nile with mud. The details are obscure but it seems probable that the king in fact used clay banks or "bunds"

The Grand Coulee Dam on the Columbia River, Washington, USA. Completed in 1942, this masonry gravity dam contains a reservoir of 11,500 Mm^3. The associated hydro-electric power station has a capacity of 1944 Megawatts (MW), to be increased by 1980 to a total of 3254 MW.

to hold river water on low-lying land when the annual flood receded. Whatever the facts of King Menes' operation, it is known that such a system has been used by peasant cultivators on the Nile's banks throughout history. So simple and so effective is this method of water conservation that even today one sixth of Egypt's cultivated land is irrigated in this way. The pharaohs are known to have gone a step further: they built canals. One pharaoh, 4000 years ago, widened and deepened the natural channel to Lake Qarun, which lies 70 km. southwest of Cairo. Five hundred years later another pharaoh built a wall around the lake, thereby increasing its capacity and providing, after the annual flood, irrigation for some 20,000 hectares of formerly unproductive land.

By 1000 B.C. the *shadoof* was well established as a means of raising water from the river to an irrigation ditch at a higher level. With the aid of this counterbalanced bucket-on-a-pole, one man could lift sufficient water each day to irrigate one tenth of a hectare (1000 m^2). Later the Archimedean screw was adapted to raise water up a 30° incline. Now two men could water three tenths of a hectare a day. Before long someone invented the *saqia*, a large wooden wheel with a series of clay pots on its rim. With one buffalo and a saqia an Egyptian farmer found he could irrigate 2 hectares each day.

Such devices were not confined to Egypt. Inventive farmers throughout the arid Middle East were developing similar gadgets. In Persia and in India, where there was abundant underground water, the bullock-operated Persian wheel became the fashion. This system of clay pots on a suspended endless fiber chain could raise water from hitherto unreachable depths.

Once the art of raising water, even if only a few meters, had been mastered, distribution was achieved by the simplest of all methods, gravity flow in open channels. Here only two problems faced the early engineer: the first was seepage, which in a long earth channel could result in the loss of a very high percentage of the water it was intended to convey; and the second was the establishment of a suitably gentle gradient along the channel, irrespective of ground undulation. To reduce seepage in naturally porous ground the simple answer was often a lining, either of clay or of cut stone slabs. The problem of gradient was usually solved without recourse to undue excavation or water bridging, by siting water channels along the general line of natural contours.

The same system—gravity flow—was used in the earliest known large-scale urban water supply undertaking. This was the remarkable network of aqueducts built by successive Roman leaders between 312 B.C. and A.D. 226 to supply the Roman capital. These aqueducts were constructed almost exclusively of cut stone blocks laid partly at or slightly below ground level, and partly on elaborate stone colonnades where they crossed low-lying land. Varying in length from the modest 16 km. of the Aqua Appia, Rome's first, to the 90-km-long Aqua Marcia, they sometimes bridged other natural watercourses, and were no mean feats of engineering. Over a 6-km. stretch approaching Rome, two aqueducts, the Aqua Marcia and Aqua Claudia, were subsequently used to carry later aqueducts on their backs; indeed, in the case of the former there were ultimately three separate water channels running one above the other. Eight of the early aqueducts had substantial raised sections, the Aqua Claudia and the Aqua Anio Novus each running for a total of 14½ km. on colonnades.

Since these aqueducts conveyed spring, river, and sometimes lake water by natural flow, they necessarily did so incessantly, and provided more than the citizens of Rome needed in their houses and in the city's public baths. The surplus was used to provide constant flushing of the city's drains, which flowed ultimately into the river Tiber. Rome thus not only had the world's first major public water supply scheme, which delivered, when completed, more than 1000 liters per head per day for a population close on 1 million (a generous supply even by modern standards), but also boasted the world's first waterborne sewage system, which worked well, but which was not to become normal practice in Europe until many centuries later.

When engineers began to convey water through tunnels and pipes they had a great advantage over earlier water-supply men, because they found that levels had no longer to be maintained throughout. All that mattered now was that the outflow from a gravity pipe system should be lower than the inflow. Between these points the pipes could follow the lie of the land, rising above the inlet point where necessary or falling below the outlet. Operating on the principle of the gravity siphon, hydrostatic pressure maintained the flow. Nor had this flow to be continuous; it could be interrupted by any convenient system of control without the water flowing over, as would happen in an open gravity flow system. Now only as much water was allowed to flow as was actually required for use.

The next significant step forward was taken with the invention of the mechanical force pump. By means of this device it became possible to force water through a pipe that had its outlet at a higher level than its inlet. In the history of water supply perhaps the most famous early use of force pumping was in the London Bridge waterwheel pumping station set up in 1581. Peter Morris, an English engineer of Dutch–German origin, was granted a 500-year lease of the space beneath the first arch at the northern end of the original London Bridge for the installation of a huge tide-operated waterwheel. This was linked to reciprocating force pumps of Morris's own design to pump water into a city conduit system. So successful was Morris's waterworks that by the middle of the 18th century his successors owned three waterwheels, installed in three arches and driving 64 small pumps delivering 7500 m^3 a day.

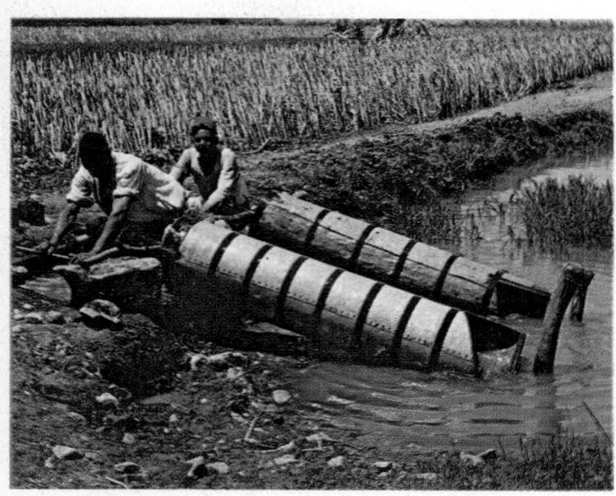

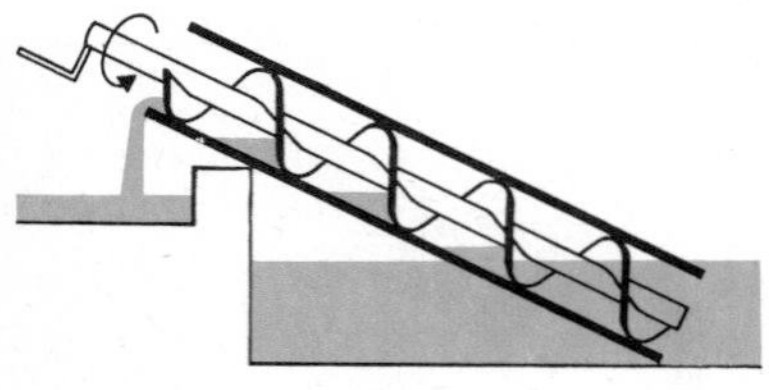

Above: the Archimedean screw. Water is carried up between the spiral paddle and the sides of a wooden cylinder. Left: Archimedean screws in use near Cairo, Egypt.

Right: the interior channel of the Roman Pont du Gard aqueduct in Provence, France.

The purpose of the earlier water-raising devices that originated in the Middle East was as simple as their mechanisms. They enabled the peasant farmer to irrigate land situated above the normal water level. And in those countries where the annual summer flood had provided water on fields above the winter river level, they made it possible for him to take a second winter crop. This was the germ of the system of perennial irrigation introduced by British civil engineers in India during the 19th century. In the main, these were run-of-the-river schemes in which barrages were built across steadily flowing rivers such as the Indus to divert part of the water into a network of distribution canals. French and Belgian engineers built a similar barrage across the Nile directly south of Cairo. While allowing the summer flood to pass over, this held back the normal steady river flow, raising its level and diverting water into three main canals sited to distribute it across the fertile delta lands that had formerly lain parched through spring and early summer. Cotton was introduced as a cash crop and, when cotton prices fell, sugar cane partly took its place. For the first time the local farmer found that the produce of his land could pay for more food than could be grown on it.

In 1882 the British took over the administration of Egypt, and British engineers set to work to provide still more water for a rising population, already totaling 7 million—far more than the

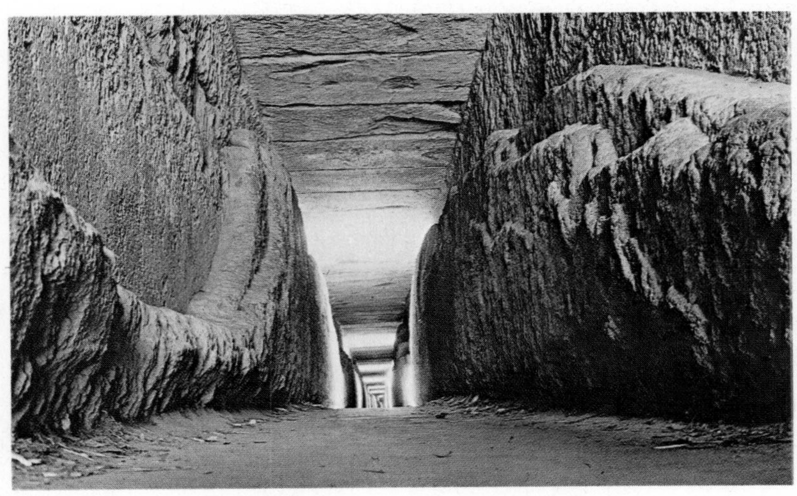

Nile had ever before nourished. The British first heightened the Cairo barrage, then decided that provision must also be made for the storage of excess Nile floodwater. By 1902 came the first Aswan Dam—a great triumph in its day, rising 27 meters above the normal water level. This dam, which was the first of its kind, had a dual role. It had to let pass the early flood, laden with its valuable silt, and then hold the clear water that followed as the flood began to subside. It was both a dam and a weir. But unlike most weirs, which do their job when the water is low, this weir had to stand up to a river in spate. A little over 3 km. long, the dam was built of 40,000 m^3 of granite block masonry, founded on the granite bedrock that lay 10 m. below the natural bed of the river. Now there was much more water to feed the canals farther north. And new canals were dug to open up new farmlands. For a decade Egypt grew steadily richer and the population soared to over 12 million.

Soon population once again began to overtake food production. The engineers took a look at their great dam and in 1912 decided to make it higher. More water was now conserved and once again Egypt's population increased. By 1933 there were 17 million mouths to feed. The engineers took a second look at their dam. This time they heightened it to nearly 40 meters, the highest they considered safe on its existing foundation. Now the reservoir could hold 5000 Mm^3 of water. Once again Egypt's growing demand was met. The Nile flood irrigated the summer crops, largely maize; and water held by the dam, released late in February, irrigated the spring crops of cotton, rice, and winter cereals. Beans and berseem (a leguminous fodder) were also planted to fix nitrogen in the hard-worked soil. Egypt became the home of the world's most intensive and skillful cropping. But in good rain years much water was still wasted, and in bad years it ran short of demand. From this fact arose the concept of overyear storage and, to some more ambitious minds who realized the danger of several bad years following each other in succession, of "century" storage. This was based on 100 years of Nile records and a somewhat uncertain theory of probability. The need for such bold planning was underlined by the still rapidly rising population. For by

1952, when Colonel Abdul Nasser came into power, it had passed the 20-million mark and 10 years later had exceeded 25 million, with the prospect of reaching 38 million by 1982. Winston Churchill had foreseen the only final solution (as indeed Napoleon had before him) when in 1899, after taking part in the British Nile campaign and learning of the original Aswan Dam plan, he wrote, ". . . and these gigantic enterprises may in their turn prove but the preliminaries of even mightier schemes until at last nearly every drop of water which drains into the whole valley of the Nile . . . shall be equally and amicably divided among the river people, and the Nile itself, flowing for 3000 miles through smiling countries, shall perish gloriously and never reach the sea."

The earliest scheme for "century" storage on the Nile in fact

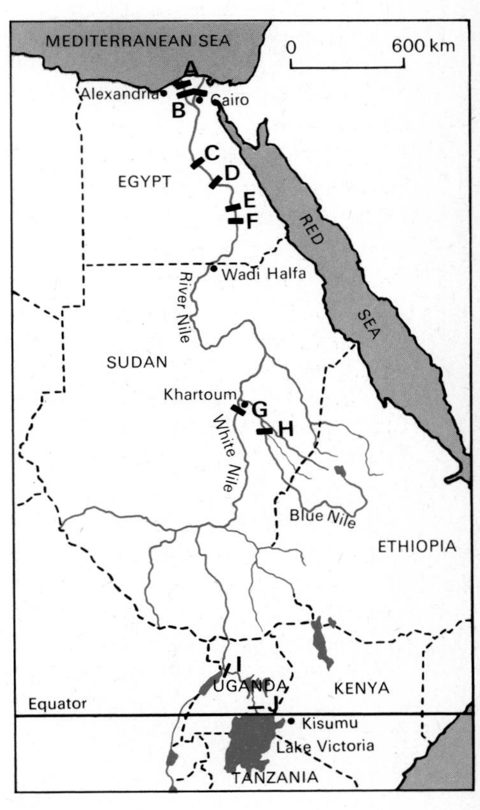

The Nile basin. The average annual precipitation at Cairo is 3 cm. and Egypt's 30 million inhabitants rely for their water supply on the annual flooding of the Nile. The average annual flow at Wadi Halfa is 83,000 Mm^3, of which Egypt uses 48,000 Mm^3 and Sudan 4000 Mm^3; 11,000 Mm^3 are lost by evaporation, and 20,000 Mm^3 flow into the Mediterranean. Any water engineering schemes must take into account the erratic flow of the Nile and make provision for overyear storage, as does the Aswan High Dam reservoir, which can contain twice the river's average annual flow. Principal control barrages are: Edfina (A), Mohammed Ali (B), Asyut (C), Nag Hammadi (D), Esna (E), Aswan High Dam (F), Gebel Awlia (G), Sennar (H), Murchison Falls (I), Owen Falls (J).

preceded the first Aswan Dam. In 1891, William Willcocks, a British engineer, proposed engineering to store water in the great lakes of the Upper Nile. The project included a main dam and reservoir at the outlet of Lake Victoria, a regulating dam at Lake Albert (through which the White Nile flows), and a storage dam and reservoir at Ethiopia's Lake Tana, source of the Blue Nile—these to be accompanied by a canal through the Sudd swamps. The Aswan High Dam project is credited, originally, to an eccentric Egyptian of Greek extraction, Adrian Daninos, today conveniently forgotten. He had perfected his plan to include a massive hydroelectric and fertilizer plant as early as 1912. In 1955 Dr. H. E. Hurst, a British engineer employed by the Egyptian Irrigation Department, advised the authorities to proceed with the High Dam project. In opposition to Anglo-American politics (which imposed conditions to which he would not agree), Nasser gave the green light to the High Dam project with financial and technical aid from Soviet Russia. The technicalities of building the Aswan High Dam will be discussed later, for it is one of the world's most remarkable engineering projects of all time, dwarfing the original Aswan Dam to an unbelievable degree, as can be seen in the diagram on page 93. But first we must examine the problems of, and the methods used in, meeting contemporary man's growing thirst for water.

Today, rivers are the basis of man's water supply almost everywhere. In the United States, where regional shortages, especially in the developing southwest, have prompted the spending of huge sums on research into alternative sources, about 75 per cent of the country's total domestic and agricultural water requirement is met by surface runoff. Elsewhere the pattern is similar, the percentage usually higher.

Diversion Barrages

The simplest method of diverting river water for man's needs is to lead the water off by gravity through an open canal or pipeline. Where the river water level varies significantly, continuous gravity feed is obtained by constructing a low barrage or weir across the river to form a constant-level intake basin.

The excess water flows over the top of the weir and continues its original course. As barrages seldom retain more than a few meters head of water, the problem of erosion caused by the overspill is a relatively minor one. However, in situations where the river is subject to a substantial summer flood, it is usual to incorporate control gates that lower the effective height of the barrage to allow the floodwater to escape more readily. In this case a concrete spillway apron is usually necessary on the downstream side to prevent flood season erosion. At the comparatively new Nangal barrage on the Sutlej River in north India, the bed of the concrete spillway apron is studded with projections to lower the water velocity before it returns to the original channel.

While the role of the dam is entirely different, its main purpose being to provide water storage, the reservoir formed behind the dam wall frequently serves as the source of a water distribution system. In this instance the intake is fed either by an open side-channel upstream of the dam or by a tunnel or large-bore pipeline leading into the reservoir below water level. In either case control gear is installed, usually in the form of hydraulically or electrically operated remote-control valves.

Often the main storage reservoir of a water supply system, if not created by the construction of a dam, must be at a higher level than the river that feeds it. There is a wide range of

Below: how a barrage is used to regulate the flow of a river to supply irrigation channels. Right: the Gudu barrage on the river Indus, India.

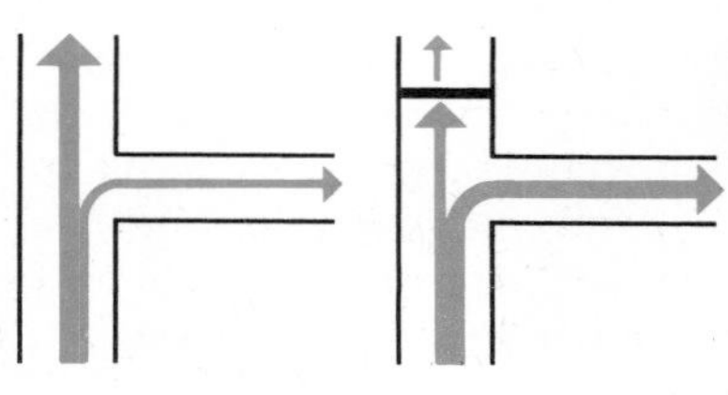

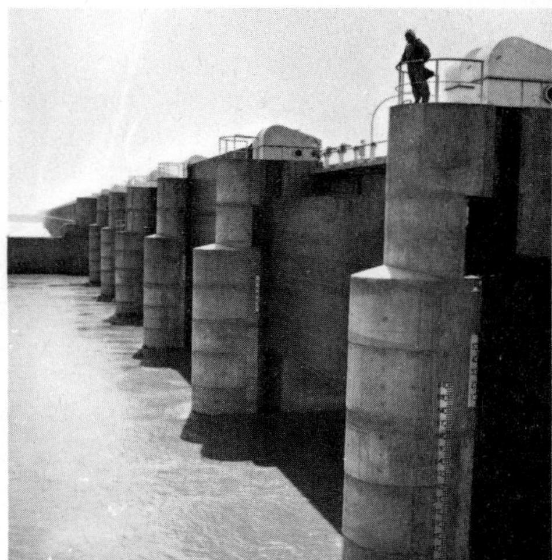

pumping plant used for raising water, the choice of basic type depending on the rate of discharge required and on the lift. Modern pumping plant is almost invariably powered by electricity and is of the impeller type. Impeller design varies from the radial flow (centrifugal) pump, which will operate against high heads but with relatively low discharge rates, to the axial flow (propeller) type, which gives high rates of delivery against low heads. Between these two extremes are various intermediate designs.

The Exploitation of Groundwater

Groundwater has been exploited in the dry Middle Eastern countries since earliest times by means of the *kanat*—a gently inclined tunnel (as much as 16 km. in length) leading up under rising ground until it is submerged by the inclined water table. Kanats are still used today in Central Asia, Morocco, and parts of the Sahara; more than 20,000 exist in Iran.

The use of groundwater as a source of supply where surface runoff is inadequate to meet demand has grown rapidly in recent years. The main method of extraction is by borehole pumping, the submersible electric pump of appropriate design for the lift that is required being used. There is a danger in groundwater usage—that of exceeding the recharge rate, when the water will fall steadily until pumping is no longer possible. This is tantamount to "mining" water. Where groundwater is intended to provide a permanent supply, extraction must obviously not exceed the recharge rate.

London's principal water lifeline has always been the River Thames, responsible for two-thirds of the total supply, though the River Lea has contributed since the middle of the 17th century. Wells and boreholes, mainly in the Lea Valley (north of the capital) and in Kent (to the southeast) provide one sixth of the current supply. However, with the city's water requirement forever rising, the time is not far distant when the Thames, the Lea, and the existing wells and boreholes will be unable to continue to meet the need, certainly not in drier summers. And today, as in so many other developed parts of the world, it is under the ground that engineers seek additional supplies. In

London, the answer to the problem, at least for the coming 20 years, has been found in the deep chalk and limestone that lies 100 km. or more beneath ground level in the Chiltern Hills, west of the metropolis. Here the Thames Conservancy has drawn up detailed plans for a network of 248 boreholes, capable of yielding 1.3 Mm^3 a day—almost exactly the average daily quantity taken from the River Thames in 1966. Already 3 test boreholes have been drilled and pumps installed. Pumping is being carried on for increasingly long periods for three consecutive summers and drawdown measurements used to check the calculated safe output of the entire network. To relate the performance of the 3 test boreholes to the 245 others still to be drilled, an analogue computer has been designed to represent the complete proposed network and is already functioning at the Water Board's headquarters.

It is 150–250 m. down in a similar 300-m.-thick limestone rock formation that one of the southeast United States' more recently discovered reserves of groundwater is to be found. This vast aquifer lies under Florida and parts of Georgia, South Carolina, and Alabama. What this source will ultimately yield is not yet known; however, natural springs and flowing artesian wells fed by this pressurized underground reservoir are already known to yield some 18 Mm^3 each day—about three times New York City's average daily consumption. Clearly the potential supply of water here is substantial.

Pumping is not the only method of exploiting groundwater. It would seem logical, since groundwater flows along impervious strata in a generally horizontal direction, that its path could be

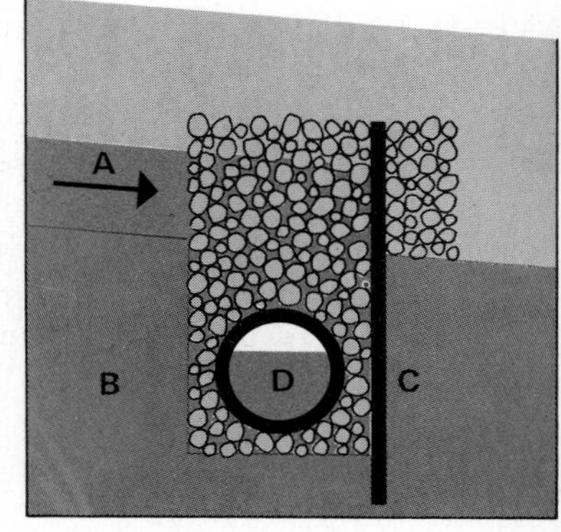

The cutoff dam at Mzima Springs, Kenya. A 4-m-wide, 650-m-long trench runs across the underground water flow (A) to a depth of 3 m. below the level of the impervious bedrock (B). A 6-m-deep steel curtain (C) laid at the downstream face of the trench diverts the water through a packing of 40-cm. boulders into the 1.2-m-diameter open-jointed concrete pipe (D).

blocked by engineering that would force the water up to form artificial springs. This is the principle of the cutoff dam, an example of which is to be found at the Mzima Springs in Kenya, where the Mombasa water supply authority has successfully used this device to add to their supply (see page 79).

Water Storage

Since the water flow in any natural source tends to fluctuate, surface water diverted directly for agricultural or urban use can never be more than a relatively small percentage of the mean annual discharge. In practice the percentage diverted in run-of-the-river schemes rarely exceeds 30 and is often less. Where a higher utilization ratio is required, provision must be made so that excess water flowing during wetter weather can be stored and supplied during subsequent dry periods. With suitable storage facilities, water utilization can be much higher and may even approach the 100 per cent mark, though 85 per cent of total flow is, in practice, a high proportion. Where utilization exceeds 50 per cent it will usually be found that there is an element of overyear storage in the scheme.

Until the middle of the 19th century, valley dams were rare and water storage was almost invariably achieved by the construction of large, shallow, open water basins contained by earth embankments. There were two reasons. A water basin was usually found to be a cheaper proposition than a valley reservoir of the same capacity; and suitable sites for embankment reservoirs were not hard to find, even near cities. Where the topography is such that a relatively large man-made lake can be formed by damming a comparatively deep and narrow valley, however, this form of bulk storage proves cheaper. The shallow bunded reservoir (i.e. enclosed by a low embankment) retains two advantages: it does not silt up as rapidly as most valley reservoirs, and expensive flood control spillways and control gear are rarely necessary.

An unusual storage reservoir was recently built at Hong Kong, where a suitable tract of land could ill be spared. This was constructed by damming the entrance to a deep sea inlet, the salt water being subsequently displaced by fresh. Another recently developed water-storage technique is the use of depleted aquifers. Water is pumped not out of, but into, the underground water-bearing strata, from which it can be recovered when required. In this way it has been found possible to achieve high storage capacity at low capital cost.

Seepage loss is accepted as inevitable in large reservoirs. But waterproofing may prove economic in smaller water-storage projects. Concrete is the material commonly used, but concrete laid thick enough to stand up to the unpredictable stresses and strains of settlement under the weight of water is expensive. A new technique is the application to the concrete surface of a thin film of polyvinyl chloride or butyl rubber. By this means the concrete used need not be of such high quality, or so thick, provided it has the necessary basic strength, because cracks caused by settlement are of no consequence. The cost saving can be considerable, especially in the case of repair to an old leaky reservoir. Reservoirs for irrigation or fire-fighting storage water are often made by applying polyvinyl chloride or butyl sheeting directly on the soil, or on a layer of sand added to the soil, of an excavated basin.

Apart from main storage, most urban supply schemes require means for local service storage. Reservoirs for this are usually covered concrete tanks designed to carry an estimated average one-day supply. Such service reservoirs are generally located on high ground—or on concrete stilts—near the area of supply, so as to provide the required pressure head in the distribution system without the necessity of pumping, except, of course, to fill the reservoir.

Transport and Distribution

While local domestic and industrial water distribution is today carried out under low pressure in piped systems, bulk transfer of water for other purposes from main storage to service storage reservoirs is more commonly by gravity flow, whether by open or closed channel. The pressure tunnel has, however, become more common of late where the natural gradient is excessive. In such a situation a gravity-flow system at atmospheric pressure creates a problem at the lower end, where water, arriving at high velocity, must be carried away to avoid a buildup of pressure in a closed system, or an overflow in open channels. There is no such problem in a pressure tunnel, because control valves can be incorporated, and where engineering can provide tunnels guaranteed not to fail under the high pressures met, and at less cost, these are clearly a better proposition.

One of the most impressive recent engineering projects involving the large-scale transport of water is the Australian Snowy Mountain scheme. Of the 130 km. of aqueducts so far completed in this scheme, upward of 30 km. are pressure tunnels, typical diameters being 6–7 m. The diagram on this page illustrates the gigantic scale of this water development and the water transport problems its designers had to face.

The Snowy Mountain scheme in New South Wales, Australia. Right: the map indicates the immensity of the project, which has three aims. First, to divert water from the Snowy River (which flows through well-watered land) across the Great Dividing Range (gray) into the Murray River, to augment the supply of water flowing through the irrigated western plains (see Snowy–Murray profile below). Secondly, to divert water from the upper reaches of the Murrumbidgee River by way of the Tumut River into the Murrumbidgee as it joins the Murray River to the northwest (off map). Tunnels, pipelines, dams, and pumping stations have been constructed in difficult mountainous terrain to divert water that originally flowed in directions (A) into directions (B). Thirdly, the scheme has provision for the generation of 2500 MW of hydroelectricity from 11 power stations. The first of these began operating in 1955, and the project, at a total estimated cost of $960 million, is expected to be complete by 1975.

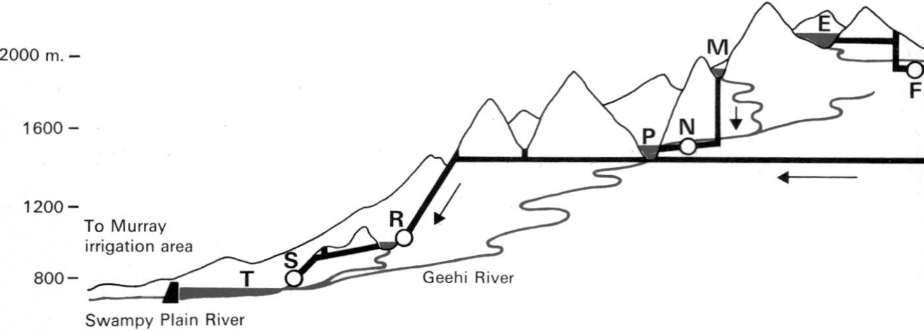

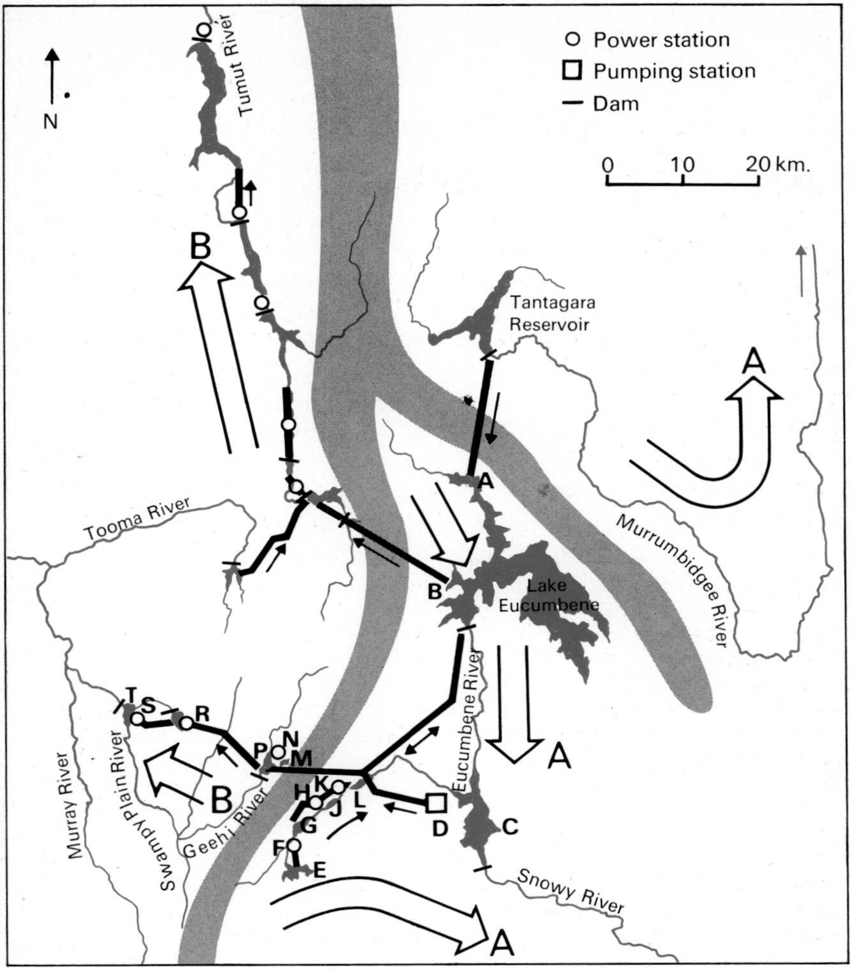

Power station
Pumping station
Dam
N
0
10
20 km.
Tumut River
Tantagara Reservoir
Tooma River
Lake Eucumbene
Murrumbidgee River
Eucumbene River
Murray River
Swampy Plain River
Geehi River
Snowy River
A
B
C
D
E
F
G
H
J
K
L
M
N
P
R
S
T

2000 m.
1600
1200
800
G
J
H
K
L
C
D
Snowy River
Eucumbene River
Lake Eucumbene
B
A

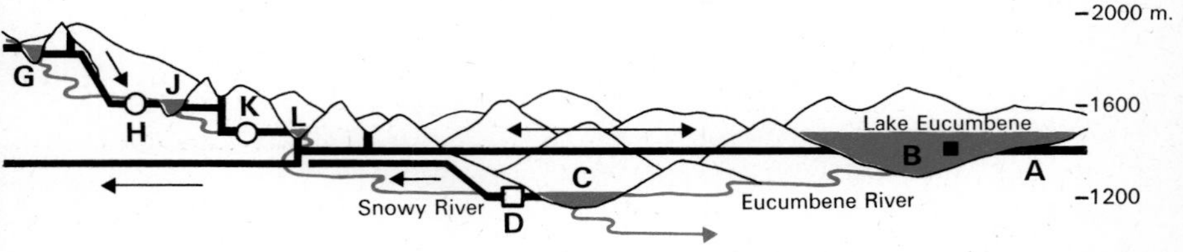

Of similar proportions is the Indus Basin Project, a joint undertaking between India and West Pakistan to regulate the flow of the Indus River system and provide all-year-round irrigation water for both countries. Six rivers join to make the Indus River in West Pakistan. The upper regions of the Ravi, Beas, and Sutlej rivers to the East pass through India and have been allocated entirely for use by India. To offset the depletion of the lower regions of these rivers in Pakistan, 400 miles of canals supply water to them from the western rivers, the Chenab, Jhelum, and Indus. Three dams have been constructed on the river Jhelum to contain a reservoir of 7250-Mm^3 capacity. The most important of these, the Mangla embankment dam, is the third largest in the world and has a hydroelectric power rating of 1000 MW.

The modern aqueduct is usually built of prefabricated large-bore concrete pipes, and experience has shown these to have a long life. The natural impurities dissolved in the water must be taken into account, as any form of corrosive action that roughens the interior surface of the pipes ultimately reduces the effective hydraulic gradient and therefore the natural flow. A feature of some modern aqueducts is the electric booster pump, installed within the water main. This can increase the natural flow in a gravity system without increasing the water pressure.

Water tunnels are usually concrete lined, not only to ensure their being watertight, but also to provide a smooth internal surface that will offer the minimum resistance to the flowing water. The 12 km. of gravity-flow aqueducts incorporated in the Snowy Mountain scheme, are mostly of rubber-ring-jointed reinforced-concrete pipes, varying in diameter from 30 cm. to 250 cm., laid in shallow trenches and covered with uncompacted soil.

The laying of water mains across rivers or other major water-courses has become quite common, and whereas formerly the method used was the expensive one of tunneling through the subaqueous rock—New York City's most recently completed 4-m-diameter water-supply pressure tunnel runs 8 km. through solid granite under the upper bay between Brooklyn and Staten Island—the newer and cheaper method is by sinking prefabricated tube sections into a prepared dredged channel, joining them, and then covering them.

The problem of large-diameter mains was not solved effectively until the very end of the 18th century, when the cast-iron pipe with spigot and socket joint was invented in England. Before this, since about A.D. 1600, wooden pipes had been widely used, though in many ways unsatisfactory. These pipes were made by boring a hole up to 20 cm. in diameter through the center of a tree trunk (usually elm or fir) by means of a horse-powered augur. The thin end of the trunk would be tapered, the thick end countersunk and banded with iron hoops. Joints were made by driving the tapered end of one pipe into the countersunk end of another. Today the reinforced prefabricated concrete pipe has provided engineers with the most satisfactory means of urban water conveyance for the largest sizes of mains, but steel, cast iron, asbestos cement, and, increasingly, plastics are used for the smaller mains.

Modern urban water distribution is complex only insofar as the pressures are concerned. As the pressure must necessarily never drop below the minimum that will provide adequate flow in every outlet in a city, and as it is both uneconomical to the supplier and annoying to the user to have water at too high a pressure, a large urban pipe network is usually divided into pressure zones, according to the distance from the nearest service reservoir, the available head, and the expected maximum volume of flow. These variables affect delivery pressure and must be taken into account in planning distribution systems.

Since it is not always possible to site service reservoirs at a sufficient elevation to supply adequate pressure throughout the area they feed, mains pressure is sometimes increased by incorporating electric pressure-booster pumps within the pipeline systems. Sometimes, too, small service reservoirs are made airtight and air is pumped into the space above the water, thus making the whole reservoir into a pneumatic pressure tank.

Irrigation Methods

Most irrigation distribution channels, large and small, in use around the world today consist of open, unlined canals. Such channels are wasteful of water, which is lost both by percolation and by the transpiration of the water-loving weeds that invariably infest the banks. Maintenance of such canals also proves costly, even where it involves only the removal of silt and weeds. By lining a canal with concrete, water losses by percolation and weed transpiration are eliminated and maintenance costs greatly reduced. Due to the higher water velocities that can be used, silting is minimal and, of course, there is no question of clearing weeds. Building a concrete lining is expensive but, again due to the higher water velocity, a lined canal designed to carry a given flow is much smaller in section than an equivalent earth channel. As a result concrete-lined canals prove economic in most situations today, so much so that elaborate equipment has been developed to mechanize their construction. A typical machine is illustrated on this page.

Maximum water velocity in unlined channels varies from $\frac{1}{2}$ m/sec in sand to 2 m/sec in clay. In lined channels, gravity-flow velocities up to 3 m/sec are not uncommon. The economies resulting from such accelerated flow can be substantial. For example, where a $1\frac{1}{2}$-m-deep unlined canal would have to be 10 m. wide at water level and 5 m. at the base, a lined channel—of the same depth and carrying the same volume of water by gravity flow—can often be designed only 3 m. wide at water level and 1 m. wide at the base.

Where concrete canal laying plant is not available, alternative materials may prove economical for lining water channels. These include asphalt, brick or tile, stabilized soil, cement mortar on mesh reinforcement, and asbestos cement. While

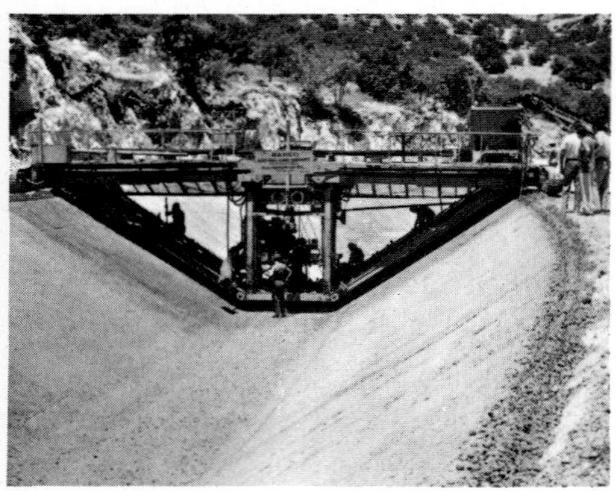

Construction techniques in water-supply engineering include the development of canal lining machines. Shown in use is one at the Jordan Canal section of Israel's National Water Carrier. Concrete is fed on to a conveyor belt and, as the machine moves forward on caterpillar tracks, an even layer of concrete 10 cm. thick is laid down.

concrete linings may be liable to damage by frost, which does not affect "flexible" asphalt and stabilized soil linings, asphalt will not stand up to such high water velocities, and stabilized soil will not resist the growth of weeds. Brick and tile linings are effective, but expensive to lay; however, where labor is cheap they may prove economically worth while.

Chapter 1 drew attention to the wastage of water in irrigation. The first step in the control of such wastage, as we have seen, is the lining of distribution channels. Once conveyance efficiency has been achieved we must take steps to minimize wastage in the fields. *Application efficiency* is defined as the percentage of the total water delivered to the land that is stored in the root zone during irrigation (the balance being lost by deep percolation, evaporation, and surface runoff). In practice application efficiency varies enormously, but 60 per cent is considered good for surface irrigation, a well-designed sprinkler system usually achieving 75 per cent. Apart from the more obvious factors affecting application efficiency, such as field gradients, excessive porosity or impermeability of the soil, and its proper preparation by the farmer, the depth of water applied at a single irrigation can be highly significant. In tests carried out on a farm in Utah, where an application efficiency of up to 90 per cent could be achieved with a 5- to 10-cm-deep application of water, efficiency was shown to drop to between 20 and 30 per cent where the depth of water applied exceeded 25 cm.

Where water available for irrigation falls short of that required for a high application efficiency, it becomes more important to know and understand the ratio of the water stored in the root zone during irrigation to the water required by the crops immediately before irrigation commences. Where water is scarce, relatively small increases in this ratio, known as the *soil storage efficiency*, have been found to double or even triple crop production.

Uniformity in the distribution of water in the root zone throughout the area of cropping is another important efficiency concept. If water is applied by surface flow from the higher boundary of a sloping field, the application efficiency will vary across the field, lowering what is termed the *distribution efficiency*. Where this ratio is low, average crop production will be low, because optimum yield will only be achieved where the water supply is just right. Yield is reduced as much by excessive water as by a shortage.

One further efficiency concept becomes important under certain conditions. This, known as the *consumptive-use efficiency*, is the ratio of normal consumption of water by the crop under cultivation to the water lost to the root zone by evaporation and deep percolation. It is normal practice to grow potatoes in ridges; but where the soil is of high permeability and the ridges well spaced, the consumptive-use efficiency of applied irrigation may drop as low as 50 per cent. Where this ratio is low in a potato field it may well be increased by eliminating the ridges and decreasing the row spacing.

There are thus many facets of irrigation efficiency, depending on as many factors. Not the least of these is the method used for distributing water over the area under cultivation. There are three basic methods: surface irrigation, by flooding or by furrow distribution; subsurface irrigation, either by exploiting natural subsoil flow or by the use of porous or open-jointed pipes under the land; and overhead irrigation, by sprinkler.

Surface irrigation by flooding is the oldest known method. The post-rainy-season flood that is a feature of the great rivers in many of the world's drier regions is used to irrigate wide stretches of the comparatively flat land often found adjoining these rivers. This system was developed thousands of years ago in parts of southern Europe, in Egypt, in the Middle East, in India, and in parts of the Far East. It is still used widely, but the

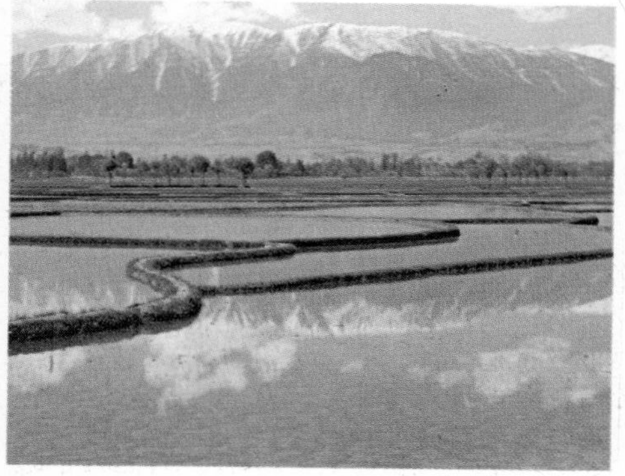

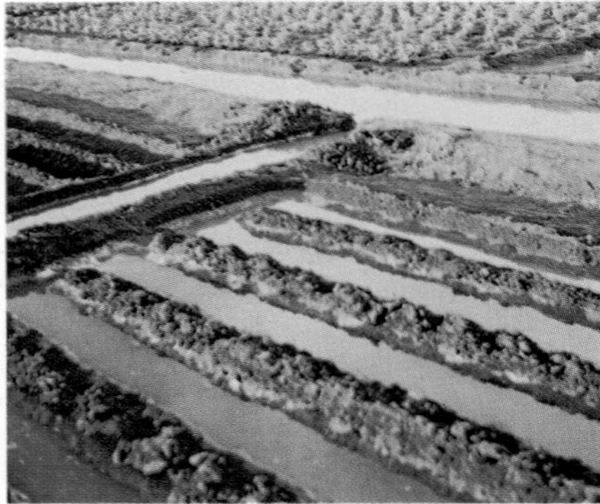

application efficiency of the method is generally low. Where the land is flat, and flooding consequently covers wide areas, there is excessive loss by both evaporation and deep percolation; and where it is not flat, there is excessive runoff. However, since irrigation by flooding is practiced traditionally in those areas where summer floodwater is abundant and therefore cheap, this may be of little consequence. More efficient methods of surface irrigation have been developed for use in areas where water, though plentiful enough, is more expensive and a higher efficiency therefore desirable.

In border-strip flooding, the fields are divided into strips varying from 10–20 m. wide, and up to several hundred meters in length. The strips are separated by low earth embankments (a height of 30 cm. would be typical) and are leveled across their width. Longitudinally they follow the land slope, the most efficient gradient being about 1:1000, though this may be increased up to as much as 1:20 where any lesser slope is impractical. Water is released into each border at the higher end from a supply ditch, and allowed to flow naturally over the surface toward the lower end. The optimum rate of water flow will depend on the nature of the soil and the length and gradient of the border, as well as on the water requirement of the crop, but it generally varies from 10 to 250 liters/sec.

Where permeability of the soil is either abnormally high or low, border flooding is unsuitable. In the former case, distribution efficiency is low. And in the latter case, percolation is so slow that application efficiency is reduced by excessive runoff at the far end. In either case the alternative is basin flooding.

Irrigation methods. Far left: basin flooding in the Vale of Kashmir. Low earth banks (bunds) *divide the fields. Left: furrow irrigation in Sudan. Crops will be planted in the earth ridges. Right: sprinkler irrigation of potatoes in Pennsylvania.*

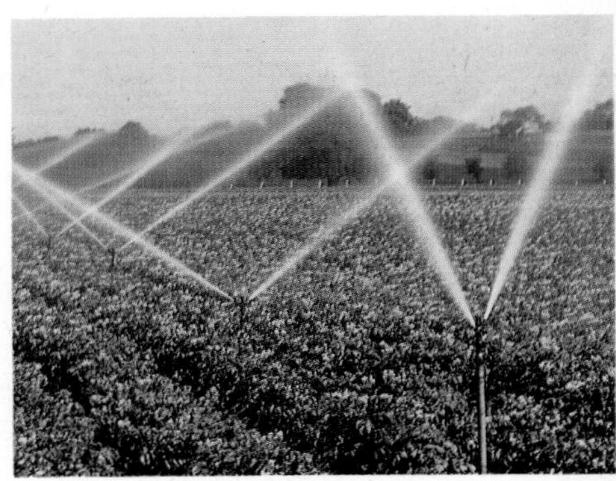

Here, in place of long narrow sloping strips, the land is divided into level basins, ideally of square shape, again separated by low embankments. Provided such basins are not too large, the optimum size depending on soil permeability, water can be made to flow all over sufficiently rapidly, even in porous soils, to ensure a reasonably high distribution efficiency. Where relatively impermeable soils are irrigated by this method the required quantity of water is let into each basin and allowed to stand as long as necessary for percolation into the soil. In hot, dry climates, however, this results in considerable evaporation loss.

Crops normally planted in rows are usually surface irrigated by the furrow method. Here the water is led between the rows, but is not allowed to wet the soil surface where the plants are located. This method reduces evaporation loss, since only a proportion (varying from 20–50 per cent) of the soil surface is wetted. It also permits cultivation sooner after irrigation. It is generally an efficient method of irrigation and is suitable for sloping as well as nearly level land. A furrow gradient of 1:100 is ideal, but slopes up to 1:10 can be irrigated by this method provided the water-flow rate is kept low and erosion checked by constant inspection and corrective action.

Occasionally, where a sandy soil is located over an impermeable layer on gently sloping land, it is possible to irrigate by natural underground flow, a system that proves highly economical. It also has the advantage that the process of irrigation at no time interferes with cultivation by farm machinery. In the Sacramento San Joaquin delta area of California, where this method has been used with great success, water is siphoned from main distribution canals into 30-cm-wide vertical-walled ditches, varying from $\frac{1}{2}$–1 m. in depth. These ditches, spaced up to 100 m. apart, provide adequate undersoil water distribution for the efficient cultivation of grain and root crops.

Subsurface irrigation can also be achieved by laying a network of porous or open-jointed pipes under the land. But this is a costly business that can rarely be justified economically, except where high-priced crops are grown and soil conditions are ideal, inhibiting downward percolation much beyond the root zone, yet permitting free lateral water movement, and encouraging upward movement by capillary action.

Under certain conditions sprinkler irrigation is more efficient than surface or subsurface methods of water distribution. Among the factors favoring it are excessive soil porosity (which makes distribution of water evenly by other methods difficult), the existence of gradients unsuitable for surface-flow systems, and the need for high application efficiency due to a general shortage of available water. In addition sprinkler irrigation has a number of special advantages, some of which may be decisive: measurement of the water used is very much easier than with other systems; sprinkler systems can be installed with little interference to existing farming operations (with surface irrigation a considerable amount of leveling is required); except for subsurface irrigation it takes less land out of production than other methods; water can, where this is desirable, be applied in small measured quantities at frequent intervals. Finally, sprinkler systems are easily used for the controlled application of liquid fertilizers in solution.

There are various types of sprinkler installation, both permanent and portable, working at pressures varying from as low as 3500 kg/m^2 to as high as 70,000 kg/m^2. The best system for a given situation depends on several factors, of which the area to be irrigated and the cost of available power are dominant. Sometimes power is not required, for some sprinkler systems will operate efficiently by gravity flow alone from a supply reservoir sited on high ground nearby.

Irrigation using seawater has been the subject of research in Israel. This has shown that many crops are tolerant to salt when grown in sandy soils affording efficient drainage. Some species will even tolerate irrigation by undiluted seawater. Hugo Boyko, as adviser to the Israeli Ministry of Agriculture, worked out the theory behind saline irrigation during a course of experiments at a farm in the Negev desert. Water percolates rapidly through the interstices of a sandy soil and these are not completely filled by plant root hairs, as is the case in silts and clays. Thus, the root hairs of crops grown in sandy soils and irrigated with seawater are immersed in saline only for the short time taken for immediate drainage to occur. The salts themselves are washed down into the lower soil layers much more effectively than in clay soils, which actually retain salt by adsorption of the sodium ion. Some of the water in the sand evaporates into the interstitial air, leaving behind precipitated salt, which is washed down by subsequent irrigation. The temperature drop at night, characteristic of all desert countries, causes condensation of this soil vapor into a supply of fresh water readily absorbed by plant root hairs.

Apart from this, some salt-tolerant crops have the ability to separate and store salt in certain of their tissues and, provided the salt concentration around their roots is not initially excessive, will actually lower it in the process. While plants cannot withstand the excessive osmotic pressure on their membranes caused by strong random concentrations of salts, they have the ability to do so when the ions in the salt solution are physiologically balanced. The ions in natural seawater are in the required ratios.

The practical result of Hugo Boyko's research is the discovery of a whole range of plants that are salt-tolerant under the right conditions. These include barley, rye, some millets (and even some strains of wheat), sugar beet, field mustard, alfalfa, some clovers, and a number of grasses and fiber-yielding plants. The significant implication is that a whole new agriculture can be developed using salt or brackish water irrigation on sandy dune lands, millions of square kilometers of which today lie barren in the world's arid and semi-arid regions.

The Engineering of Dams

In describing the methods of supplying domestic water, I omitted one important link in the chain—that of purification. But, as this will be discussed separately in Chapter 7, there remains only one major topic to deal with here—a topic common to the supply of water for domestic use, industry, and agriculture. This is the most expensive of all man's inventions in the field of water—the dam. First we must see, briefly, how dams are designed, how they differ, and how they are built.

The purpose of a dam is clear; it is a structure designed to hold back a substantial volume of water, usually in a river valley, thus forming an artificial lake or reservoir. Dams are of two fundamental types, *gravity* and *wall*. While both have to withstand the immense pressure of the water in the lake that forms behind them, the gravity dam depends on sheer weight to prevent deformation and bodily movement, whereas the wall dam is designed as a stiff membrane that, while its inherent strength resists deformation, transfers the pressure of the water to the floor or sides (or both) of the valley it blocks. In practice many dams combine both principles.

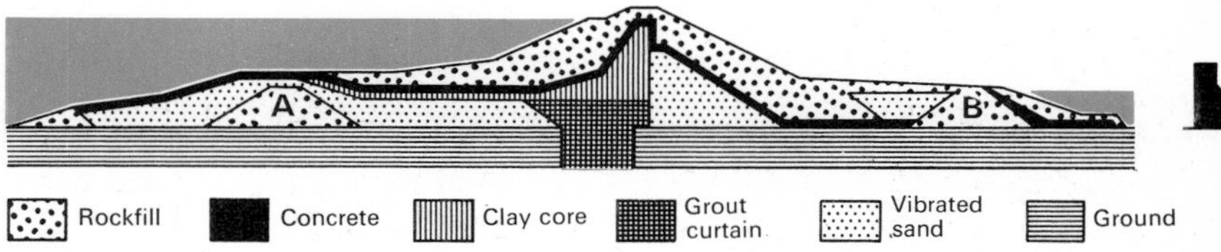

Above: cross section of the Aswan High Dam on the river Nile, Egypt. This rockfill embankment dam, 1.2 km. wide, incorporates the upstream (A) and downstream (B) cofferdams. The grout curtain (not shown completely) extends to a depth one and a half times the height of the central dam ridge. Water levels shown are maximal, and at the extreme right is a scale cross section of the old Aswan Dam. Below: the Aswan High Dam under construction, January 1967. The spillways and hydroelectric power station (2100-MW capacity) are to the left of the main dam structure.

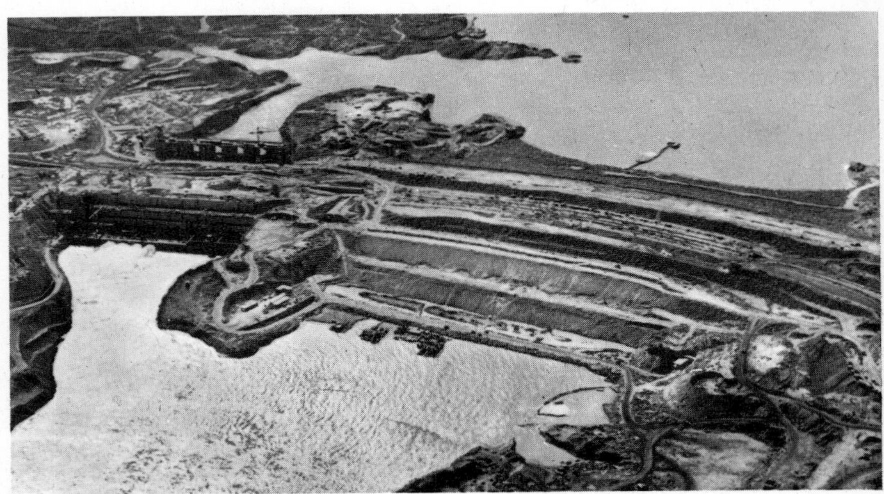

The simplest and oldest form of gravity dam, the embankment, differs from all others in that it is basically flexible, being made up of particles, large or small, that can move in relation to each other, thus giving it some of the properties of a viscous fluid. It depends for its success in holding back water on its permeability being low enough to slow internal percolation until the velocity of the seeping water is below that which would give rise to internal erosion. In practice a flexible impermeable layer, of clay for instance, is usually incorporated in it, with the purpose of arresting seepage completely. Often it is given a stone block facing on the reservoir side to help control surface erosion.

The rigid gravity dam consists of a heavy monolithic block of impervious material. While early dams of this type were generally constructed of masonry blocks cemented together, the contemporary version is almost invariably built of mass concrete.

If a wall is subjected to pressure from one side it will tend to bow and will be subject to both compressive and tensile stresses within its fabric. And as masonry and concrete are inherently weak in tension the tensile stresses induced in a wall dam must either be taken care of by suitable design, which may include reinforcement or buttressing, or be eliminated by building the wall in the form of a horizontal arch. Wall dams are therefore of three distinct types—arch, buttress, and reinforced. The most basic form of arch dam is the simple, vertical, constant-radius cylinder. This is particularly suited to the steep-sided gorge, where it provides maximum strength with the minimum volume of concrete; it is also used in the shallower V-shaped valley, where it sometimes proves to be an equally economical form.

Where the central portion of a large arch dam is unusually high in proportion to the length of its rim—a not uncommon situation in the wide, deep valley with gently sloping sides—the tensile stresses near the center of the foot of the dam wall may become excessive. This is especially likely where the wall is keyed deeply into bedrock and functions partly as a cantilever out of the ground. To withstand such high tensile stresses the wall is designed with vertical as well as horizontal curvature, like part of an eggshell. This form is known as the double curvature arch (cupola), and by designing it with its center of gravity as close to the upstream edge of its foundation as is safe, its own dead weight provides the entire structure with a measure of prestress, putting into compression that part of the wall where the water pressure will tend to induce tension, and thus greatly increasing its strength.

Stress analysis of the arch dam wall, especially the double curvature arch, can be a time-consuming process; and while the computer is being increasingly used to speed this necessary operation, structural models are frequently used. Such a model, usually of a mixture of plaster of paris and fuller's earth, is built accurately to scale and is fitted with electric strain gauges at points where the maximum stresses are likely to occur. Pressure is now applied to the upstream face of the model, usually by using mercury confined in a large fabric bag, and the strains are measured. The strain-gauge readings, scaled up, give the designer a clear picture of how the full-size dam wall will function in practice. Such model testing is not unduly expensive, and provides the designer with an economic means of trying out alternative dam wall shapes.

The tensile forces induced by the pressure of the water in a straight wall dam can be taken care of in two ways. The simplest method is by buttressing the wall at frequent intervals along its length. Provided the distance between the buttresses is not too great, the tensile stresses that occur in the sections of wall between them can be kept within the limits imposed by the material of which it is constructed.

The alternative method is by incorporating steel reinforcement. Until the development of modern systems of prestressing, reinforced concrete was uneconomic for dam walls because so much expensive steel was needed to obtain the required tensile strength. Today, by prestressing the reinforcement (in tension) so as to induce in the concrete around it a compressive stress exceeding the maximum tension it must subsequently withstand, a wall can be constructed with a quarter of the steel. The buttress dam was pioneered in the United States as a

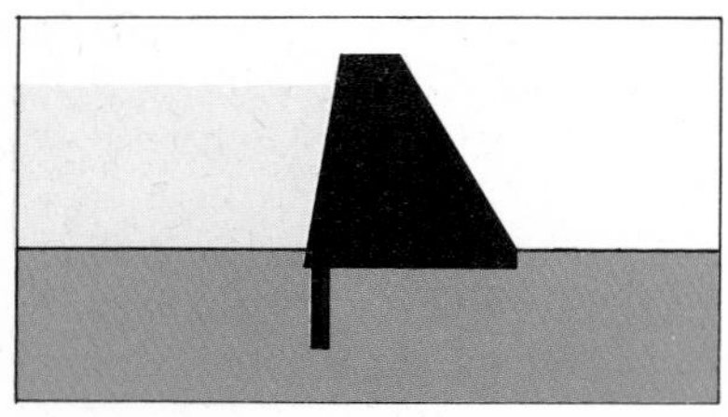

Left: cross section of a solid gravity dam, which resists hydrostatic pressure by sheer weight. Modern examples of this type of dam are usually constructed in mass concrete, unlike the masonry block design of the Grand Coulee Dam (see page 68).

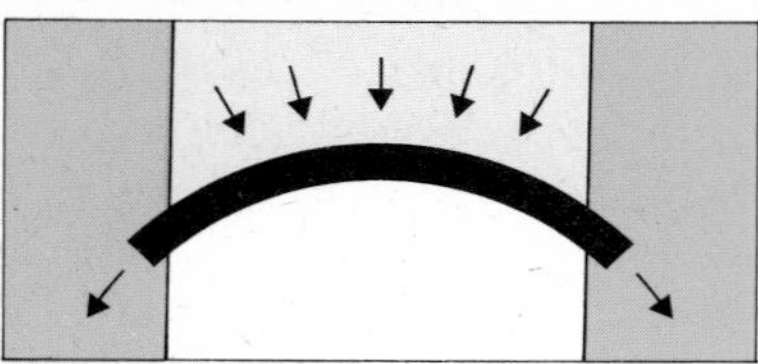

Left: a constant-radius arch that derives stability from the opposing compressive and tensile forces in the shape and by distribution of load to abutments. Right: control dam at Long Sault on the St. Lawrence Seaway.

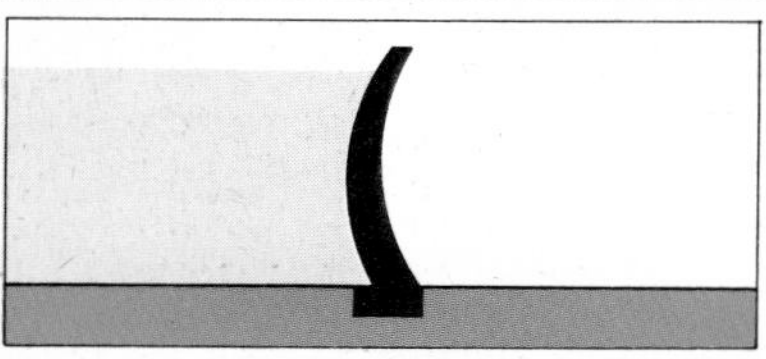

Left: cross section of a double curvature (cupola) dam (plan as above). Curvature in both horizontal and vertical planes confers greater pressure resistance to the wall. The Kariba Dam combines the cupola and solid gravity designs.

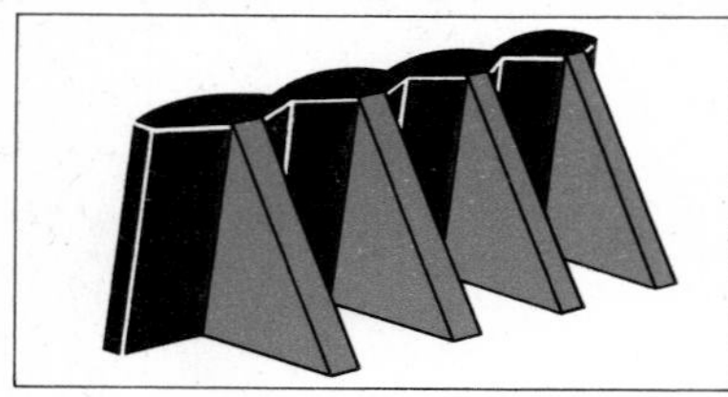

Left: the buttress principle. This design is used in long straight dams, combining economy of concrete with good stability. Each section, with its buttress, acts as a gravity dam. Near right: Lawers Dam built for the South of Scotland Electricity Board.

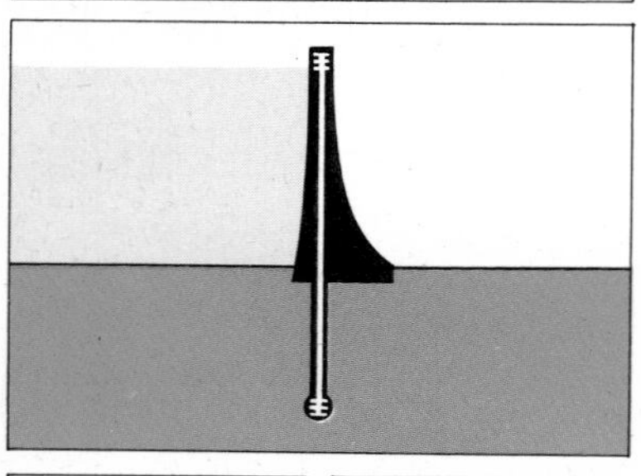

Left: prestressed reinforced design. Steel cables are set in the dam wall and anchored in the foundations. These are stressed in tension to induce compression in the concrete, and confer stability to the wall by cantilever action at the base. Right: prestressed dam under construction in Switzerland.

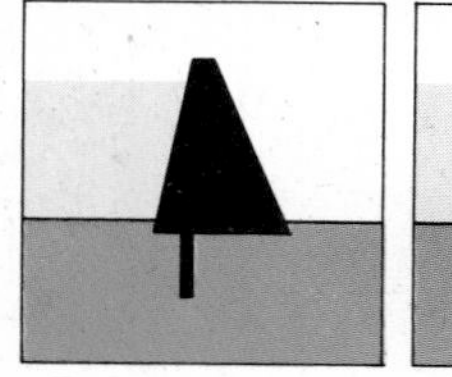

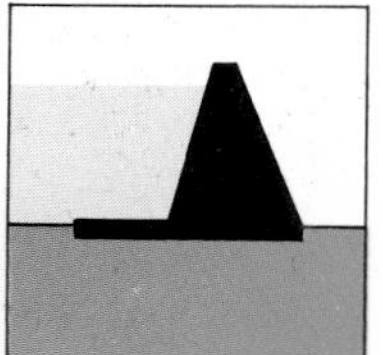

Two methods of reducing underdam seepage. Far left: a cutoff curtain—an impervious layer (usually grout) slotted into the foundation. Near left: an apron—an impervious layer laid horizontally in front of the upstream face.

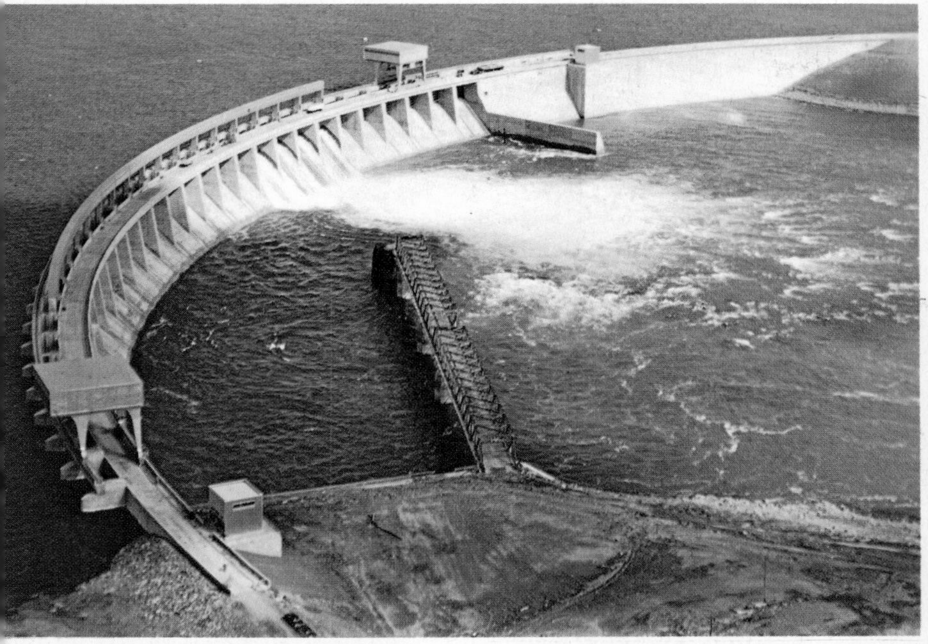

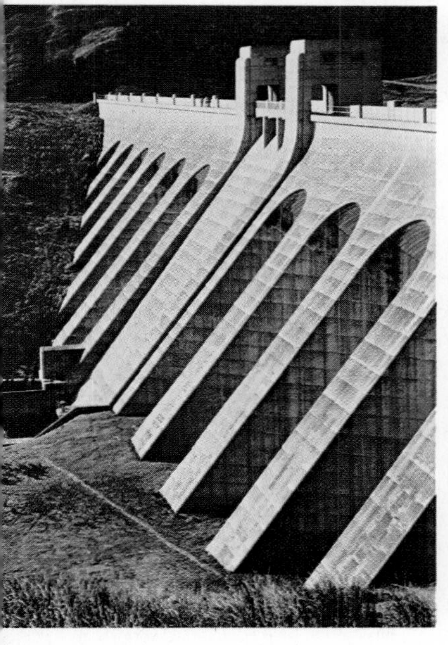

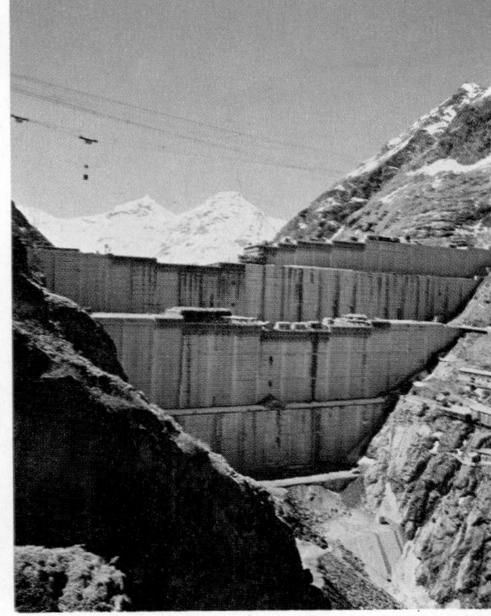

means of minimizing the total mass of concrete required to hold back a given volume of water. The same aim was pursued in Europe by building cellular or hollow gravity dams. That a gravity dam can be made lighter without reducing its capacity to withstand water pressure may seem anomalous; to understand why this is possible we must take a brief look at the theory of hydraulic pressure and its effect on dam foundations.

Dam Foundations

The principle of foundation work generally is that of spreading the load until the pressure per square meter falls below the bearing strength of the natural stratum that supports the structure. Where dams are founded on bedrock, as the majority are, the need to spread the load is rarely critical and the foot of the dam wall, bearing directly on the rock beneath it, need only be as thick as is necessary for vertical stability. In the case of the 25-m-high Medlow Dam, New South Wales, Australia, the 3-m-wide base of the wall is just twice the thickness of its top.

Far more significant in dam foundation design is the hydraulic pressure that may build up under the dam, due to water seepage. This pressure, which tends to lift the dam wall bodily upward, is due to a simple principle, that the internal pressure in any fluid is transmitted uniformly in all directions through the fluid. In a dam, this results, if there is the least seepage under the wall, in an upward pressure that acts to lift the wall bodily off its foundation. One cubic meter of water weighs 1000 kg. The pressure at the bed of a 100-m-deep reservoir is therefore 100,000 kg/m^2. If the base of a dam wall holding back this depth of water is 200 m. long and 100 m. wide (i.e. base area 20,000 m^2), and water at a pressure of 100,000 kg/m^2 seeps between this base and the bedrock, the total upward pressure on the base of the dam comes to 2000 million kg. But if the same dam wall has a narrow base, measuring 200 m. long but only 10 m. wide, the maximum upward pressure is 200 million kg., one tenth of the former figure. A narrow base may thus make possible the saving of many millions of kilograms of concrete. So do measures that prevent seepage.

The engineer uses several means to minimize underdam

seepage, the two most important being the *cutoff curtain* and the *apron*. The former consists of an impermeable curtain slotted deep into the bedrock on which the dam is founded. The principle of the curtain is to so lengthen the path of possible underground seepage, and so increase the resistance to seepage along that path, that the hydraulic pressure drops to an insignificant level by the time any seeping water reaches the point of danger under the dam wall.

The apron is a similar device, comprising an impervious layer laid horizontally in front of the toe of the dam wall. It acts in the same way, by lengthening the possible seepage path. Both cutoff curtains and aprons are usually constructed of high-quality waterproof concrete and are monolithic, as far as possible, with the concrete of the dam wall. Sometimes steel-sheet piling is used for a cutoff curtain, being driven deep into the valley bed and then keyed into the concrete of the dam wall built later above it. Another method is by pumping cement grout under pressure into a series of boreholes driven downward into the formation on which the dam is to be founded. High pressure forces the grout into any fissures in the bedrock, forming an impervious layer within the rock on setting. A comparatively recent technique, which has been used extensively on the foundations of the Aswan High Dam, is vibration. Sand can be compacted so completely by suitable vibration that it forms an all but solid rock, the particles of sand being shaken down thoroughly so that virtually no air- or water-filled interstices remain between them.

Spillways and Erosion Control

An important feature of almost every dam is a spillway designed to permit the escape of excess water during times of flood. Essential in any dam, it is particularly vital in the case of a nonrigid embankment dam, which could be seriously scoured, and possibly completely breached, by uncontrolled water pouring over the top. There are three main types of spillway: the first releases the excess water over the top of the dam wall; the second allows it to run into an overflow shaft leading from a point within the reservoir; the third diverts the excess water to a side channel or tunnel leading beyond the end of the dam wall. Sometimes excess water is released through gated apertures in the dam wall: the Kariba Dam has such apertures 30 m. below high-water level.

In a concrete dam an overfall spillway consists usually of a section of the main dam wall where its rim has been kept lower than elsewhere or where control gear can lower its effective height at will. Typical control gear are drum gates (which are made to rise by their own buoyancy—water being let into the drum from the reservoir side to lower them, or let out on the opposite side to raise them again), and mechanically raised sector gates.

The shaft spillway consists of a large-section concrete pipe that passes through the dam wall and up to the reservoir surface at some point behind it. The mouth of such a spillway is usually flared like a bell.

In the side channel spillway a weir, with its associated control gear, is located some distance back from the dam wall on the reservoir side; excess water flowing over it is led by open channel or tunnel around the end of the dam. This has the advantage that the dam wall can be of uninterrupted design. Also it avoids the possibility of the dam's foundation suffering erosion from the excess water pouring down an overfall spillway, and eliminates the problem of adequately leak-proofing the point where a shaft spillway pierces the wall.

Whatever the method selected for releasing excess water, the engineer must somewhere face the problem of safely dissipating the energy of the escaping water. In times of flood this unwanted energy may run to several hundred million watts. In an overfall spillway, millions of kilograms of water may fall uninterrupted over the dam wall, possibly gouging out a great hollow below and ultimately endangering the dam's foundation. This problem is usually investigated by the use of scale hydraulic models in which various shapes and profiles of stilling basin are tested. The Grand Coulee Dam, which harnesses the Columbia River in the United States, has a "bucket" profile on the downstream side, designed to ensure that the downward rush of surplus water is turned back over itself, thus dissipating its energy harmlessly on the special concrete of the bucket. The designing of this bucket was not as simple as it may look to the layman; its profile had to be exactly right so that it would turn over the rushing water at high as well as low flow rates. It was evolved by testing a series of possible shapes in an accurate scale model of the proposed spillway and its outflow channel.

When a scale model of the spillway of an arch dam at Coues, France, was hydraulically tested, it was discovered that at certain flow rates the falling water developed vibrations that considerably increased its destructive power at the lower point of impact below the downstream face of the dam wall. This vibration could not have been anticipated; but it was easily eliminated by building water dividers along the spillway crest. Had the vibrations not been forestalled on the actual dam, serious damage might have been done to the foundations.

Dam Construction

The first task in designing a dam is to select the site. This means finding the spot where the optimum retention of water within existing geographical, social, and political limits will

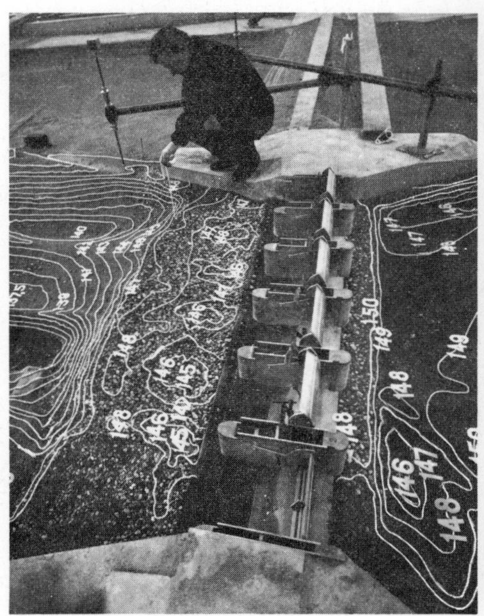

Scale models of projected water-engineering schemes are tested in the laboratory to determine the behavior of the finished construction. Here, in the hydraulic laboratory at Chatou, France, engineers are studying water flow and its effect on the topography of the channel around the Gerstheim barrage on the Rhine.

result in the most economical construction. It involves a geological survey of the ground on which the dam is to be founded, not only to ensure that it can support the weight of the dam itself, but also to provide the designer with the information he needs to design foundations that will remain impervious to the head of water the dam will create. It involves detailed physical, geographical, and social surveys (possibly a zoological survey too), so that the area to be inundated by the artificial lake that will be formed can be accurately mapped and all the resulting implications handled. It involves a survey of the labor and transport problems likely to be encountered at the proposed site. In remote areas it may well be necessary to build a road, a railway, or perhaps an aerial ropeway, to handle the enormous quantities of cement, stone, and rock that will require moving, and to bring in earth-moving and concrete-making plant and other heavy machinery. It may require the construction of an entire township, complete with hospitals, entertainment facilities, and other amenities, to house the labor force.

Dams, by their very nature, are built across natural watercourses, and the engineer's first problem is to divert the normal flow of water from the site while the dam and its foundations are being built. This will usually involve the design and construction of one or more cofferdams, and the digging of alternative channels or sometimes of tunnels. The cofferdam is a temporary dam designed to exclude water from the site of the permanent engineering work. Sometimes the cofferdam is subsequently incorporated in the main dam wall. Alternatively it may later be removed, or possibly left on the upstream side to be submerged as the water level rises behind the finished dam. It is sometimes a comparatively simple engineering construction, such as an encircling wall of interlocking steel-sheet piling driven into the river bed. For extra strength it may be a double wall of sheet piling into which clay is packed. Or it may be more substantial. In the Kariba Dam, the upstream cofferdam comprised a semicircular wall of mass concrete, 13 m. high × 2 m. thick, founded on a 6-m-wide foundation taken down to bedrock (see page 105). This was designed to hold back the river and divert its dry-season flow, partly through a tunnel driven in the right bank and partly via an open channel excavated in the riverbed between blocks of the main dam foundation. When the summer flood came, the water was allowed to flow over the cofferdam and the partly completed foundation work of the main dam wall until the rainy season was over; when the water level had fallen sufficiently, the remaining water was pumped out of the foundation area and work resumed. This cofferdam remains deeply submerged on the upstream side of the completed dam.

In the case of the Rance estuary tidal power station, of which I shall say more in Chapter 5, a huge encircling cofferdam had to be built in tidal water. To achieve this a series of 19-m-diameter cylinders made up of 40 cm. × 1 cm. interlocking sheet steel piling were placed along the line of the cofferdam and filled with sand. The gaps between these cylinders were then bridged with short double arcs of piles, the enclosed area again being filled with sand. To minimize leakage, frogmen packed clay bags around the base of each cylinder.

The cofferdams used in the construction of the Aswan High Dam were designed as part of the final huge embankment and themselves consisted of rockfill embankments, each almost as high as the old Aswan main dam. These were concreted over and the water pumped out from between them. The main dam foundation, consisting of a cement grout curtain down to bed-rock, was built between the cofferdams, the river flowing through six great diversion tunnels driven through the granite on the eastern side of the gorge. Over the foundation was laid a waterproof core made of clay, behind which, on the down-stream side, was an embankment of sand compacted by vibration. More compacted sand was laid between the upstream cofferdam and the core, and the final profile was made up with granite rockfill cut from the sides of the river valley. Finally a "toe" was laid upstream of the southern cofferdam, again with a rockfill embankment at its farthest tip, the gap being made up with compacted sand. Concrete was used as a sealing layer over the upstream face of the main dam, the layer running on between the vibrated sand and rockfill on the north side.

When cement sets by its chemical action with water, heat is

released; and where a large mass of concrete is involved, the temperature rise can be considerable and it may take months for the concrete to cool right through. As the concrete cools it contracts; and the result is that construction joints tend to open. Unless special precautions are taken, the result, in a large dam wall, is the formation of serious cracks, which result in a weak structure that may not be watertight.

One or more of three steps are taken to overcome this problem. First, the concrete is laid in alternate blocks, usually 15–30 m. wide. This series of blocks is allowed to cure for several weeks before the gaps are filled. The second procedure is to cast flexible sealing strips—usually of copper, though cheaper materials are also used—into the concrete near the upstream face so that they form bridges across each vertical construction joint. Pipes are also sometimes cast into the concrete so that cement grout may subsequently be pumped into the cracks that will still form, inevitably, between adjacent concrete blocks. The third procedure is to provide artificial cooling for the concrete. There are two methods, and sometimes both are used. The first—precooling—is achieved by chilling the coarse aggregate or the water, or both, before the concrete is mixed and poured. Much of the heat of hydration may then be absorbed by the cold concrete mixture acquiring normal temperature. The second method is achieved by laying pipes between each pour of concrete, through which chilled water is circulated until the excess heat has all been piped away.

In dam building, excavation and the dumping of many millions of kilograms of spoil (soil plus rock and gravel) often form a major part of the contract. One of the principal tasks in the construction of the huge Kuibyshev Dam across the Volga in the USSR consisted of dry and wet excavation. One quarter of this 5½-km. barrier is a concrete weir with a shipping lock at one end; another quarter is a concrete power house. Of the remaining 2¾ km., half is blocked by a natural island, the other half by a simple earth embankment founded on sandy clay. The excavating machinery used—reported to be one of the largest collections ever assembled at one spot—included one 1000-ton electric monster powered by 8000-kW motors and

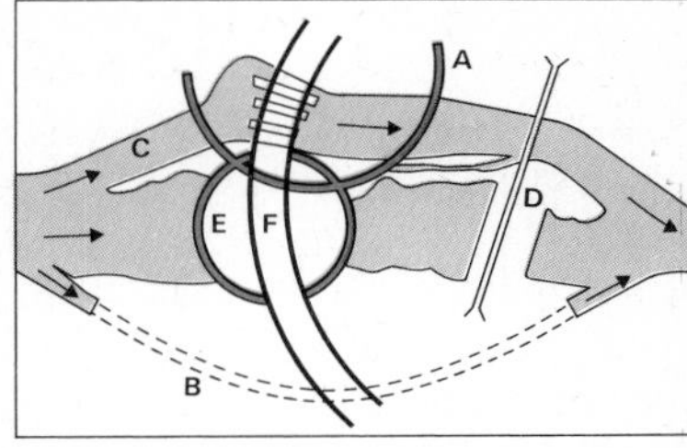

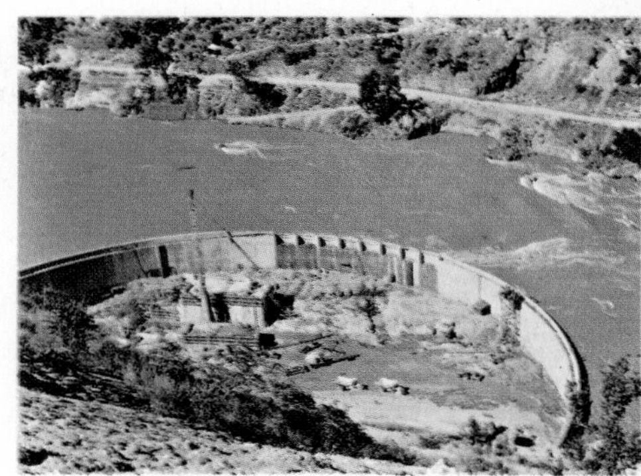

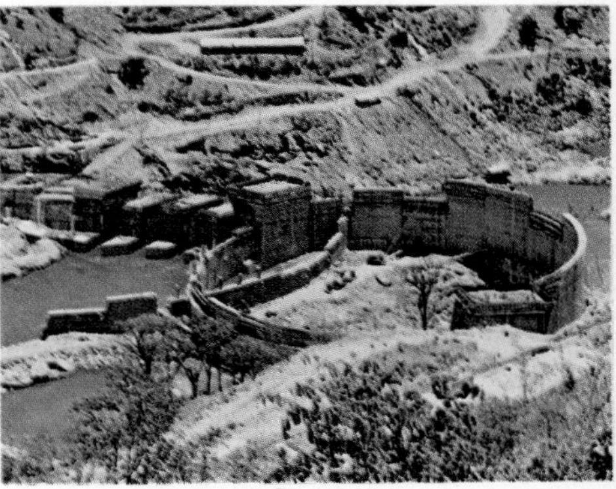

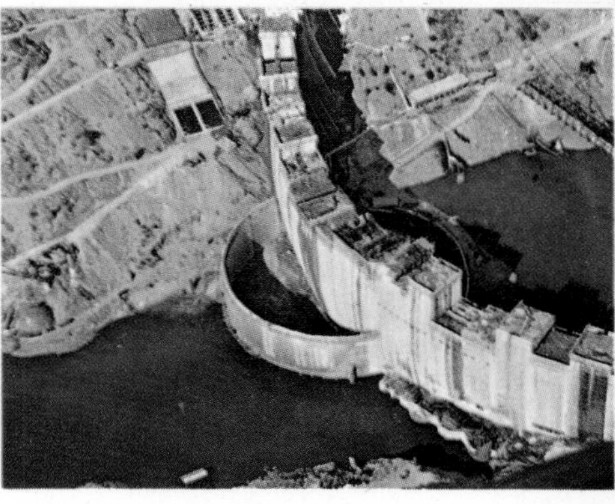

Stages in the construction of the Kariba Dam. The diagram (above) is a condensation of several time stages. Phase 1: the left-bank semicircular cofferdam (A) and the diversion tunnel (B) were built simultaneously. A diversion channel (C) was dug, and blocks of the main dam laid down in the cofferdam. Phase 2: the river was dammed downstream with rockfill (D) and the walls of cofferdam (A) dynamited to effect complete diversion of the water. The main circular cofferdam (E) was constructed. Phase 3: cofferdam (E) was pumped dry and the main dam (F) started. Phase 4: the diversion tunnel and channel were sealed and the main dam completed. Top: Phase 1, March 1957. Center: Phase 2, November 1957. Bottom: Phase 3, November 1958. The project was completed in February 1960.

capable of shifting 20,000 m^3 each hour. The machines dumped the mud they lifted to form the central section of the huge earthen embankment, which today withstands the water pressure of Europe's largest man-made lake, measuring 490 km. long by 40 km. wide.

There are other problems, some substantial, some less vital, that may have to be attended to in any large dam project. The Kuibyshev Dam blocked a waterway used as a major transport artery; so it was necessary, as at the other four major hydroelectric and irrigation complexes on the Volga, for the dam to be bypassed by a canal with locks. Indeed these canals were in each case built first so that shipping would not be interrupted by the subsequent construction work. They have made possible winter as well as summer shipping on the Volga, since the abundant electrical energy available permits the heating of the canals so as to prevent ice formation, icebreakers maintaining channels through the ice that forms on the huge man-made lakes. Sometimes, as in many of the hydroelectric projects in Scotland, which are sited on salmon runs, it is

Some world dams in order of reservoir capacity. The Mangla Dam, one of three containing the Mangla Reservoir, is the third largest dam in the world.

Dam	Type	River	Country	Reservoir Capacity Thous. of Mm^3	Hydroelectric Output (MW)	Year completed
Kariba	Concrete Gravity/Cupola	Zambesi	Rhodesia	185	600/1500	1959
Bratsk	Concrete Gravity	Angara	USSR	179	4500	1963
Aswan High	Rockfill Embankment	Nile	Egypt	160	2100	Under Construction
Krasnoyarsk	Concrete Gravity	Yenisei	USSR	107	6000	1967
Sanmen Gorge	–	Yellow	China	66	1100	1960
Hoover	Concrete Gravity/Arch	Colorado	USA	37	1340	1936
Glen Canyon	Concrete Arch	Colorado	USA	35	900	Under Construction
Volgograd	Concrete Gravity	Volga	USSR	32	2400	1961
Grand Coulee	Masonry Gravity	Columbia	USA	11.5	1944/3254	1942
Mangla	Earthfill Embankment	Jhelum	West Pakistan	7	1000	1967

necessary to provide water "ladders" during and after the construction of dams, to enable migratory fish to reach their traditional breeding grounds.

And finally there are sometimes political, social, and even zoological, problems that require solution. The Kariba Dam across the Zambezi River has created an artificial lake 280 km. long and up to 32 km. wide, partly in Zambia, partly in Rhodesia. The social problem was the resettlement, by two different civil authorities, of the entire 50,000-strong primitive and superstitious Batonga tribe, former inhabitants of a 5000-km^2 fertile area in the river valley. Added to this was a zoological riddle, for many thousands of wild animals were driven from the artificial lake area by the rising waters, seriously disturbing the balance of local ecology. And in place of the animals a huge new freshwater fish population grew up encouraged by the sudden appearance of mile upon mile of still water choked with submerged vegetation. So zoologists, biologists, botanists, and doctors all had to watch for repercussions.

Political problems originated in the fact that the Zambezi rises in Angola, discharges into the Indian Ocean in Mozambique, and meanwhile flows along borders of Zambia, Rhodesia, Botswana, and South West Africa, all of which, along with Malawi and South Africa, claim an interest in the river. Economically Kariba was essentially a straightforward capital project, for the companies operating the Zambian copper mines required a sizable and steady source of electrical power, were prepared to pay for it, and were able to persuade the World Bank to help finance it.

How different from that of Kariba was the problem Colonel Nasser had to face in securing finance for the High Dam. Scheduled originally to cost \$1.2 million million, it was estimated that this project would add \$900 million to Egypt's annual national income, but would probably never produce any direct revenue. No wonder that its value came to be measured more in terms of expanding political ideology than in ready cash, and that its whole conception became an exercise in political philosophy as much as an engineering challenge.

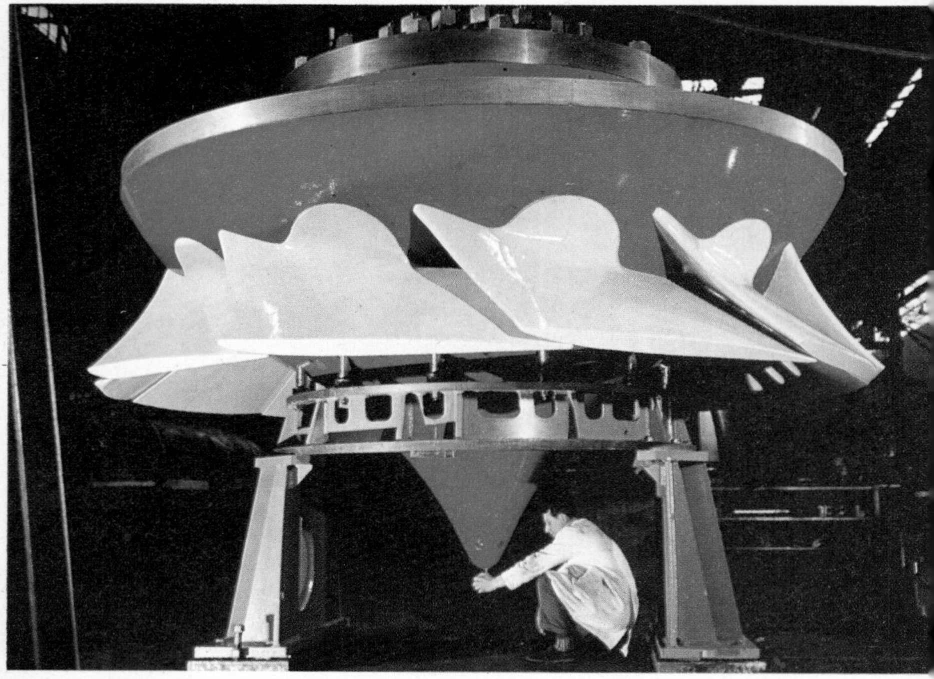

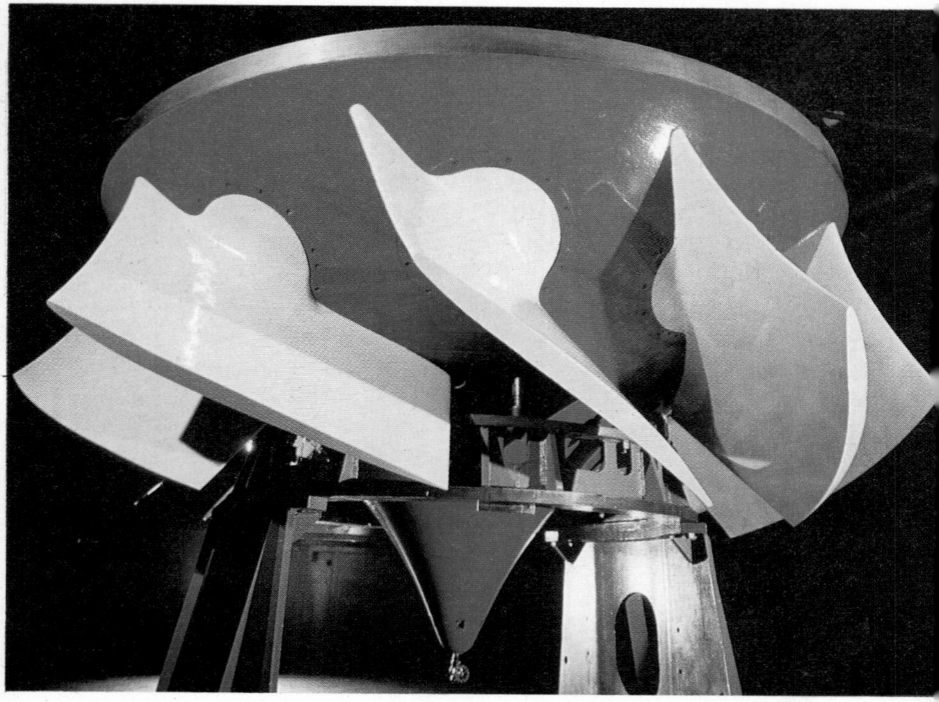

5 Hydroelectricity

At the Munich Exhibition of 1882 the world's first demonstration of hydroelectric power took place almost unnoticed. A little-known engineer, Schukert by name, displayed an electric motor that apparently ran without batteries. In fact Schukert had installed a similar motor on the bank of the river Isar at Hirscham, 9½ kilometers away. This motor, driven by a waterwheel, acted as a generator, the current being led to the motor at the exhibition by copper cable.

The waterwheel had been used for untold centuries to convert the energy of moving water directly into mechanical power, and by the early 19th century engineers had developed waterwheel designs of high efficiency. A pair of overshot waterwheels installed at a cotton mill at Catrine, Scotland, in 1824 operated from a 16-m. head of water with an efficiency of 75 per cent, delivering 500 horsepower. Each wheel was 16 m. in diameter and 3.5 m. wide; and though they turned at only three revolutions per minute, these wheels were successfully geared to operate spindles rotating at no less than 9000 rpm.

The Deriaz-type reversible pump-turbine, designed and built by The English Electric Company Ltd. for the 225-MW. Valdecanas pumped-storage hydroelectric scheme completed in 1965 as the first stage of Spain's hydropower development program. Closed (top) and open (bottom) positions of the fully-adjustable turbine blades.

Before we take a look at contemporary water-turbine design, the relationship between energy and power, and the mathematical concept of pressure "head" in water perhaps need some elucidation. The "head" of a particular volume of water is the potential energy stored within it by virtue of its elevation. This can be converted to kinetic energy (the energy of motion) by letting the water flow to a lower level. It is expressed in terms of height. Imagine 1000 kg. of water in a tank at the top of a tower. Any mass falling freely under the action of gravity accelerates at a rate of 9.8 m/sec^2 and falls 4.9 m. in the first second of free fall from rest.

To measure energy we use the joule, 1 J being the energy required to give a mass of 1 kg. an acceleration of 1 m/sec^2 over a distance of 1 m. Suppose our 1000 kg. of water is released from the tank at the rate of 10 kg/sec. Falling under the action of gravity, each 10 kg. of water therefore acquires a kinetic energy of $10 \times 9.8 = 98$ J in each meter of free fall, or $98 \times 4.9 = 480$ J/sec, which represents 480 watts (W) of power. It is this energy of motion that can be converted into mechanical energy by routing the falling water through a waterwheel or turbine. A modern turbine linked directly to a generator operating at a combined efficiency of 85 per cent will convert our 480 J of kinetic energy into 408 W of electrical power. Our example concerned the energy output of 10 kg. of water falling under the action of gravity: 100 kg. of falling water would produce 10 times the power output, and 10,000 kg. would yield 1000 times the power.

Water-Turbine Design

In practice the water led to a modern turbine does not fall freely, for it is conveyed through pipelines and is fed to the turbines either in the form of a high-velocity jet at atmospheric pressure, or as a moving body of enclosed water under pressure. For the jet the energy output is a function of the velocity of the water flowing. This is the principle of the *impulse turbine*. In the enclosed turbine the principle of hydraulic pressure is in operation. If the surface of the supply reservoir is 100 m. above a pressure turbine, the latter is said to be working at a head of

100 m. Here the energy output of the water flowing through the turbine is not dependent on its velocity. The variable with which we are chiefly concerned is, in this case, the operating pressure. With greater heads less water need flow for a given power output. Conversely, the same power output can be obtained with a turbine passing a large volume of water at a relatively low head. Turbines operating on this principle are known as *reaction turbines.*

The early impulse turbine, with flat vanes, had an efficiency of 40 per cent. The curved vanes introduced later avoided uncontrolled splash and the consequent energy wastage, and raised the efficiency to 65 per cent. In 1889 an American, Lester A. Pelton, patented an impulse turbine that had divided, curved buckets designed to split the jet in two, with half the water acting on each side. This design, known as the *Pelton wheel* (see page 112), had an efficiency of 80 per cent, a figure that has subsequently been raised to 90 per cent by further improvements in the jet nozzle and in the shape of the buckets. The Pelton wheel is most efficient where the pressure head is high, giving the jet a correspondingly high velocity. Modern versions, using two, four, and sometimes six jets to a single wheel, are common today in high-head power stations such as that at Reisseck, Austria (1750-m. head). The lower limit of head for efficient Pelton wheel operation cannot be precisely defined since it varies with the volume of water available. However, there are many small Pelton wheels in service around the world at sites where the head is 200 m. or even less. Control of these wheels, by either deflecting the jet or reducing the nozzle aperture, is a simple matter. Moreover, they give an efficient output over a wide variation in load.

More than a century before the early impulse turbines were developed, a device known as *Barker's mill* had been invented in England. This worked on the principle of the modern rotating lawn-sprinkler. Water was fed under pressure into the axle of a wheel on which a pair of jets were mounted tangentially in opposing directions. This first known reaction turbine was extremely inefficient and it was not until 1827 that a new design was developed by a Frenchman, Fourneyron. In this outward-

The Pelton wheel (impulse) turbine. Right top: water volume is controlled by a needle valve in each supply nozzle, and the jet is symmetrically divided at each bucket of the runner. Right bottom: inspecting a completed runner. The cutout profile at the tip of each bucket facilitates water flow.

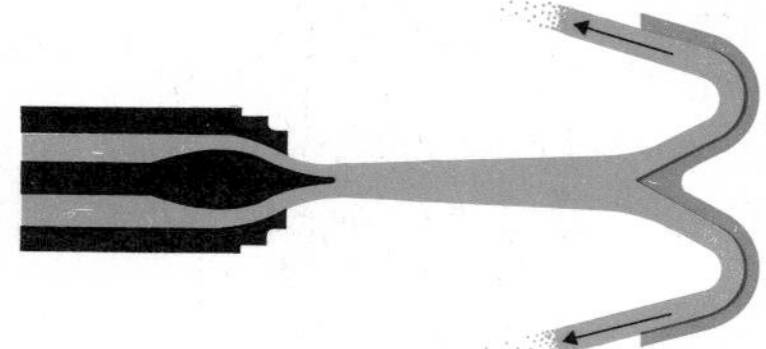

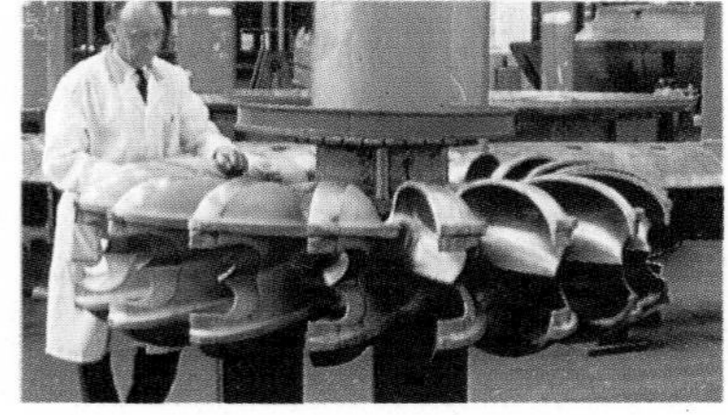

The Kaplan (reaction) turbine. The diagram is a cross section of a typical low-head installation incorporating a vertical Kaplan turbine/generator unit. The volute chamber is formed in square-section concrete and is fed directly from the reservoir. Fine control of the pitch of the turbine blades makes Kaplan units efficient over a wide range of heads, particularly those of only a few meters.

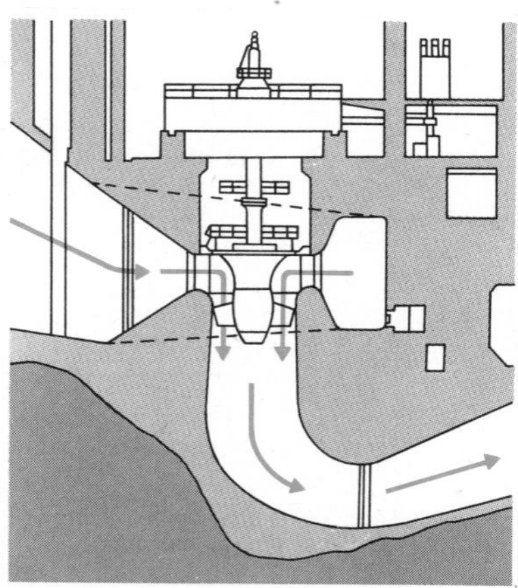

Right: a Kaplan turbine runner is lowered into place at the Priest Rapids hydroelectric power station (946 MW) on the Columbia River, Washington.

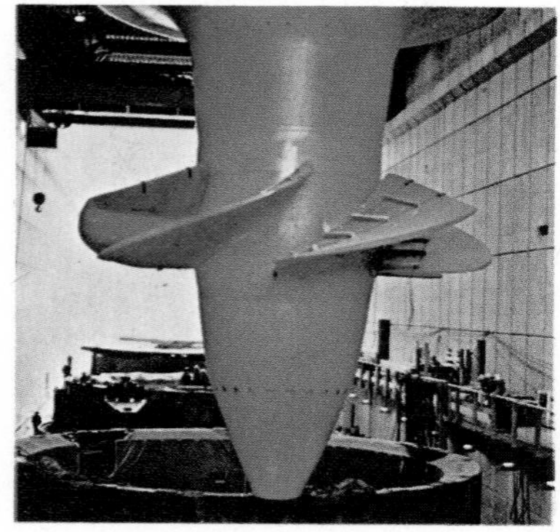

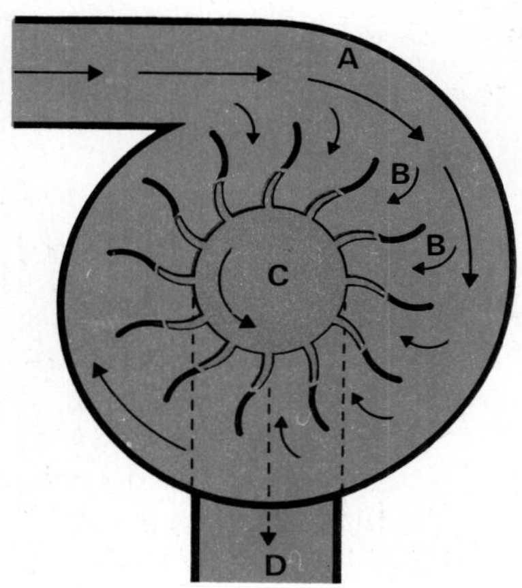

A plan of the water flow in the Francis (reaction) turbine. Water under pressure completely fills the volute chamber (A), and is deflected by adjustable guide-vanes (B) onto the blades of the rotating runner (C). The water flows away vertically beneath the runner into the tailrace (D).

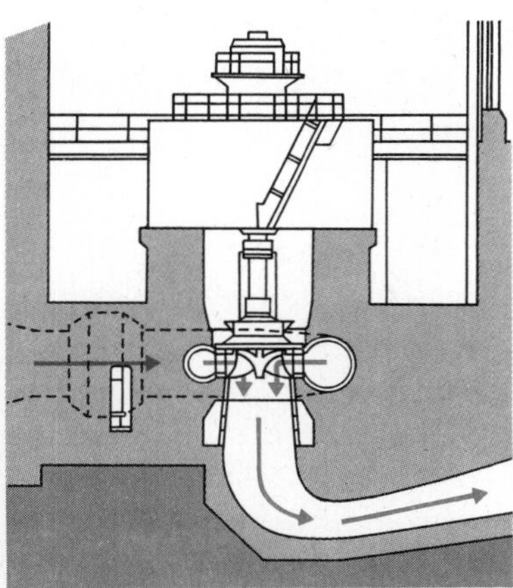

Cross section of vertical Francis turbine/generator unit in a high-head installation. Water reaches the turbine through steel pressure pipes and by way of a circular-section steel volute chamber. Below: detail of water flow at turbine runner.

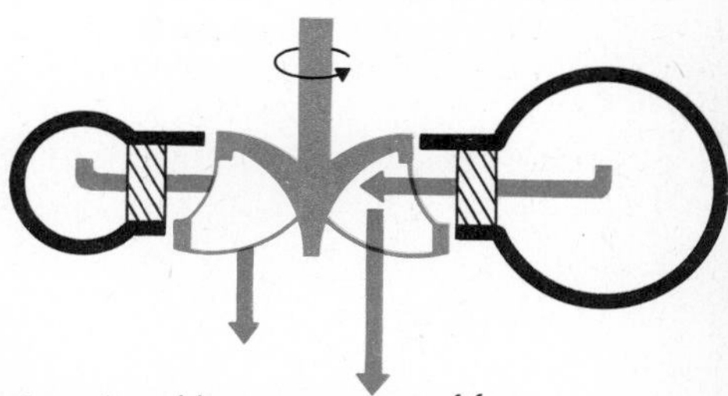

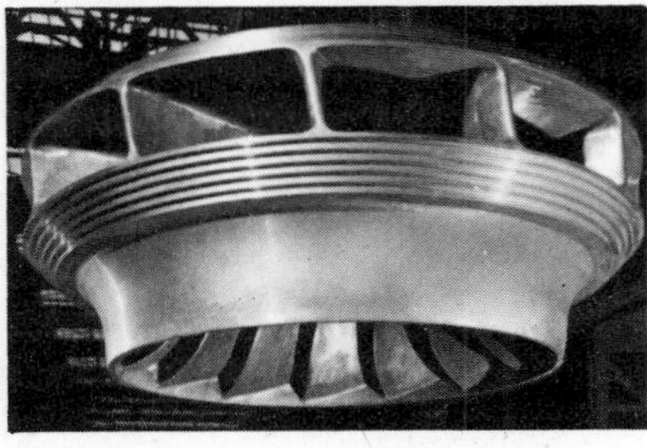

Francis turbine runner; one of four installed at the Ffestiniog pumped-storage scheme, North Wales *(see page 122)**.*

flow turbine the water was fed, under pressure, into the center of a ring of fixed deflector vanes, which diverted the water radially outward onto the vanes of a rotating runner. An efficiency of 75 per cent was achieved, but the device was not easy to regulate. The design soon gave way to the inward-flow turbine, invented in 1855 by an American, J. B. Francis. In the *Francis turbine* the water is led, under pressure, through a steel volute chamber (rather like a huge snail's shell) onto the fixed outer ring of curved guide vanes that direct it onto the curved vanes of the centrally rotating runner. The shape of these vanes is critical in the turbine's efficiency and it was a British engineer, James Thompson, who invented a system of adjustable vanes, which provided a greatly increased measure of control. The Francis turbine is widely used today in power stations operating at heads varying from 30 m. to 1000 m. It can achieve an efficiency of well over 90 per cent under optimum conditions, but this falls off rapidly as the load is increased or decreased.

It was not until 1913 that there was any significant further development in the design of turbines. This time it was a Czech,

A sectional model of a 39,000-hp. twin-jet Pelton turbine designed to operate at a head of 396 m. at 428 rpm.

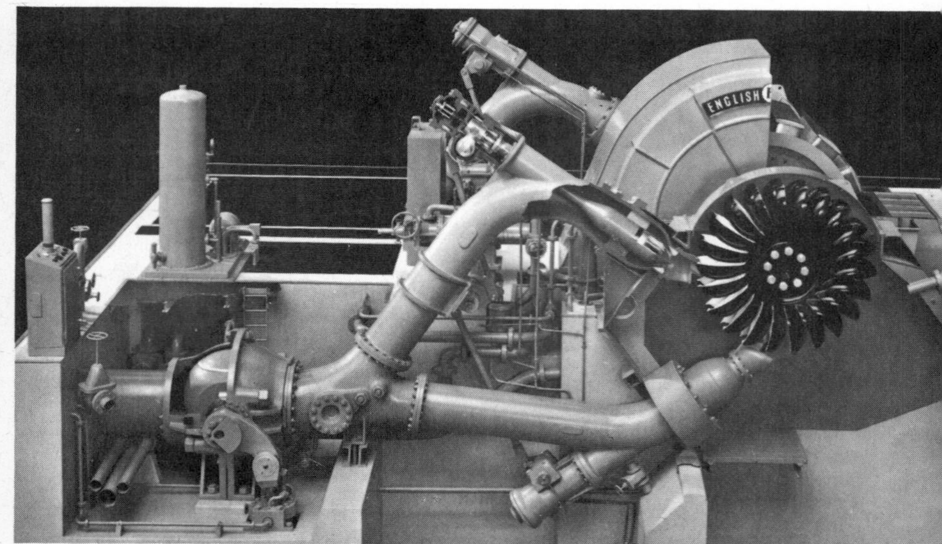

Kaplan, who patented a reaction turbine of entirely new design. In the *Kaplan turbine* the water, under pressure, flows parallel to the axis of the machine, turning a runner that has blades similar to those of a ship's propeller. The pitch of these blades, like those of the guide vanes past which the water first flows, can be adjusted or "feathered" like those of an aircraft's propeller, while the turbine is actually running. In this way the turbine can be adjusted not only for highest efficiency over a range of operating heads, but also in response to sudden variations in load. In the modern Kaplan turbine the pitch of the blades is controlled automatically by a governor. Although the Kaplan turbine is never quite as efficient as the Francis at optimum head and load, an efficiency of 90 per cent can be assured over a relatively wide range of head and load, and its efficiency at low heads is considerably greater. It is being used increasingly in power stations where the available head of water is 50 m. or less.

A recent variation of the Kaplan turbine is the *bulb generator*, in which the alternator is housed horizontally in a steel pod suspended in the water, the runner being at one end of the pod.

Construction of a steel volute chamber suitable for medium- or high-head Kaplan or Francis turbine installations.

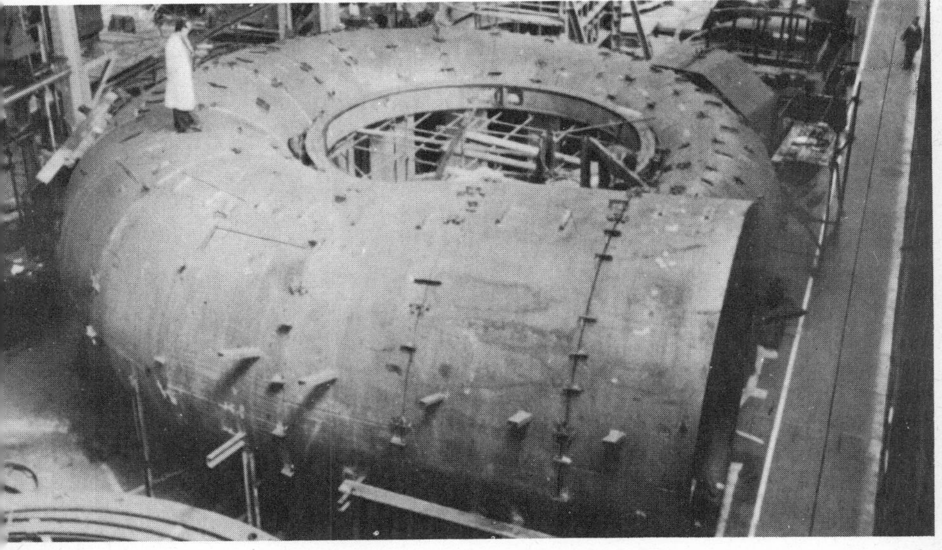

This design is suited to situations where the head is so low that it is impractical to arrange the water intake vertically above the *tail race*, the water outlet channel. Developed in France, this is the form of generator used in the world's first commercial tidal power station on the river Rance near Saint-Malo in France (see page 129) and in the recently completed low-head power station on the river Rhone at Pierre-Bénite, near Lyons. The latter installation has four of the largest bulb generators yet constructed, each delivering 20 MW with a head of only 7.95 m. and a flow of 330 m^3/sec. These units are 5.2 m. in diameter at the widest point, the runners having a diameter of 6.1 m. By using this pattern of turbine at Pierre-Bénite, Electricité de France saved themselves \$4¾ million, half on account of the simpler civil engineering works, and \$600,000 on each generator, the extra amount comparable Kaplan units would have cost to manufacture.

The Flexibility of Hydroelectric Power

Of the various forms of energy available to man the potential energy of water is the most convenient for conversion into power. In the heat engines that work by steam and internal combustion, we have the problem of obtaining and transporting fuel. We have to convert the latent energy of that fuel into heat by combustion, and then to convert the heat into mechanical energy. Often the mechanical energy must be stored, requiring a further conversion process into electrical energy. There are the waste products of the combustion stage to dispose of: some of these are solid, some partly gaseous. In every step power is inevitably wasted. The overall efficiency of a modern steam-powered turbine rarely exceeds 35 per cent, and of one powered by a gas engine 25 per cent. The modern diesel engine does a little better, achieving an efficiency of 45 per cent. The development of nuclear power production has eliminated the problem of transporting large quantities of fuel. One gram of uranium 235, destroyed by fission in 24 hours, produces 1000 kW of power throughout the 24 hours. To obtain this much power from coal during the same period 36,000 kg. would have to be burned. The nuclear power station does not pollute the air with its waste products, for no smoke or gas is produced. But it has created a new problem: that of the occasional disposal of spent radioactive fuel.

Water power, by contrast, has many advantages. There is no fuel problem at all, no waste products of any kind to dispose of. The involvement of heat ends with the natural process of evaporation by the sun and the upward movement of water-laden air due to convection, caused again by the sun's heat. The subsequent energy conversion process is extremely simple, the acquired potential energy of the water being converted by gravity into kinetic energy, by the turbine into mechanical energy, and by direct coupling to a generator into electrical energy. Modern generators achieve efficiencies as high as 95 per cent. Coupled to a turbine operating at 90 per cent efficiency this provides a machine that converts about 85 per cent of the water's available potential energy into electricity. Control, too, is simple and the response to control immediate. In a steam-powered plant there is a very considerable delay in bringing the generators from rest to high power—that is, the time taken to produce the required steam. The same is even more true of the nuclear power station, in which it may take hours or even days to bring a reactor core to the point when the fission chain reaction begins. A hydroelectric generator can be switched on

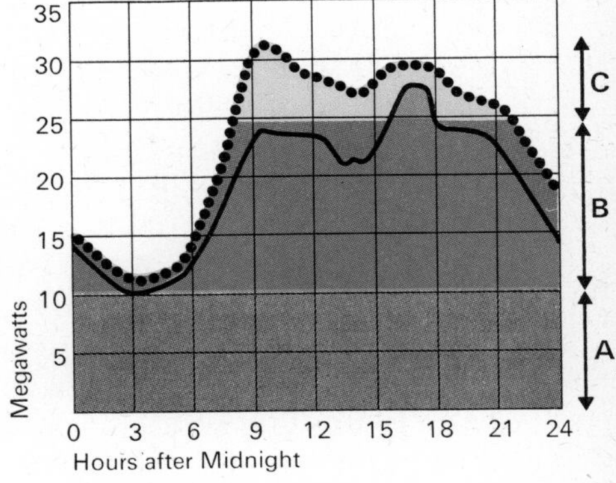

Electricity-demand pattern for 24 hours. A constant base load of 10 MW (gray) is provided by large coal-fired, oil-fired, or nuclear power stations (A). On a typical winter day (solid line) anticipated load fluctuations (green) are met by medium-sized conventional or hydroelectric power plants (B). The evening peak (blue) is met by diesel generators or hydro-electricity plants (C). On a very cold day (dotted line) plant B operates at full capacity a little longer (green and orange) and extra demand (yellow) is met by standby plant (C).

in the time it takes to open the water intake control gates—perhaps two minutes, possibly less.

It is a mistake to think of hydroelectric schemes only in terms of high-pressure heads. In recent years the development of low-head turbines has progressed so dramatically, especially in France, that today engineers can use a large volume of water at a low head almost as efficiently as a smaller volume at high head. In practice the local topography usually dictates what pressure head can be made available. At Reisseck in Austria a relatively low dam near the edge of a plateau is used to store water that is then conveyed by pipeline to a power station situated 1750 m. below at the foot of an adjoining valley. This arrangement gives an immense power output per kilogram of water flowing (water enters the turbines at a pressure exceeding 1,500,000 kg/m^2), but poses the problem of building a pipeline capable of withstanding the extremely high pressure. At the other extreme we find the new power station on the river Rhone operating with high efficiency at a head of only eight meters.

The production of water power has one disadvantage—that of the uncertainty of the water supply. This depends entirely on local hydrology: on the incidence of rainfall, or on the output, perhaps, of a spring. The Zambezi River in central Africa is, like the Nile, notorious for its unpredictability, quite apart from the extremely wide variation of its flow throughout the normal seasons. It was partly to create a good working head, but primarily to provide a huge storage reservoir, that the Kariba Dam was built 130 m. high. This reservoir, 280 km. long and with a storage capacity of 185,000 Mm^3, provides a steady flow of water throughout the year, making possible an uninterrupted power output of 600 MW. This will be 1500 MW when the second stage of the power station is completed early in the 1970s.

One of the major problems of electric power supply is the constantly changing pattern of demand. To meet these huge and sometimes rapid fluctuations in demand, power supply systems must be capable of rapid alterations in output. Of the three basic types of power station in use today, the nuclear-powered plant is the least flexible. It takes literally days to bring a nuclear reactor up to full power output, and if power is to be produced economically from a nuclear reactor, output must remain virtually constant. The only method of reducing power temporarily at a nuclear power plant is to let steam run to waste. This expedient would defeat the entire object of nuclear power production, which is to produce electricity at low cost. This applies also, though to a lesser degree, to conventional coal-fired and oil-fired plant. Here power output can certainly be adjusted more rapidly, though not always as quickly as the sudden surges in demand that occur, for example, when an evening TV program of universal popularity ends and millions of housewives rush to the kitchen to make coffee. Where conventional power stations have to vary output widely through the course of a single day, economy suffers and the cost of the current produced rises. Steam cannot be generated instantaneously, and the period during which a reserve of high-pressure steam is built up in anticipation of a sharp rise in demand represents power wasted.

The hydroelectric power plant, by comparison, is extremely flexible. A trickle of water will keep the turbine and alternator spinning when the load is low, and it takes only seconds, or at most a minute or two, to open the water intake and bring the output up to its maximum. Shutting down is equally rapid. Also, negligible energy is wasted in the process of turning on or shutting down power.

Predictable variations in demand and supply are normally handled by dividing the load into two components. The first, the base load, is generally equal to the minimum demand occurring daily in the particular season. This load, which remains constant throughout the day and night, is normally met by large-capacity modern oil- or coal-fired power stations, or by nuclear power stations, which can produce a constant output at the most economic price. The expected daily surges above base load are met by other, generally smaller, conventional power plants that are brought on or off power probably once in each 24 hours, or by major hydroelectric stations. There remain the short duration peak surges, sometimes unpredictable, which require plant that can respond to variations in load rapidly and without wastage of energy. One type of plant used for this purpose is the small diesel-electric generator. This can be kept ticking over when a surge is anticipated, and even started rapidly from rest when necessary. But if a supply of water at a suitable head is available, the hydroelectric plant is usually much more suited to this role, and certainly more economical.

The flexibility of hydroelectric power is such that it can be used economically for all three components of demand, provided, of course, that the required head and volume of water is available. It is not necessary for the minimum flow to be sufficient to meet peak demand. Provided the average flow is adequate to meet the average demand and provided a reservoir can be constructed to store sufficient water to meet the surges in demand when the natural runoff drops below the required supply, then the plant can be designed to provide base loads as well as daily variations and peak load requirements—and all three at a competitive price. This applies to the Kariba power station which today provides all the power required in the Zambian copper belt.

Large-Scale Storage of Power

With the rapidly increasing demand for electricity during the past 50 years, engineers began to realize that a time would come when conventional means, including hydroelectric power, would be inadequate to supply the growing daily increases in load above base. The advent of nuclear power has, at least for some centuries, removed the immediate anxiety caused by the world's rapidly dwindling resources of coal, oil, and natural gas. Although millions of terawatts of energy still go to waste, all around the world, in the form of unharnessed or only partially harnessed rivers, suitable unexploited hydroelectric sites were often situated too far from the areas of rapidly growing demand to make transmission of the potentially available power an economic undertaking, even where it was technically feasible. The engineers realized that if they could devise means of storing electricity on a really large scale, it would be possible to increase the output of base-load power stations above the actual base load of an area, the excess generated during the low periods of daily demand being stored temporarily and put back into the system as soon as the demand rose above the normal output. Several methods of large-scale storage of electrical energy have been investigated in recent years. And since it would clearly be impractical to think of storing surplus energy generated, for example, during the summer, for use during the following winter, all work has concentrated on schemes intended to iron out the daily fluctuations in demand.

In theory there are two completely distinct ways of storing electrical energy: the direct storage of electricity itself; or the conversion of electricity into an alternative form of energy that can be stored and subsequently reconverted when electricity is required. Direct storage of electricity is possible in three ways: by the electrochemical action of galvanic or electrolytic cells, in capacitors, or by confining a high-intensity flowing current in a superconductor loop. Indirect methods include the conversion of electricity into either potential energy or heat. Heat can conveniently be stored in large blocks or bricks, beds of ceramic pebbles, or base metal nitrates. Potential energy storage is feasible using compressed air, which is easily reconverted by feeding it to gas turbines coupled to alternators, or by pumping water to a higher level. Of the more practical methods of large-scale electrical storage, water plays a major part in two; and it so happens that these two are currently those that appear most promising commercially. They are pumped water storage, which is already being used increasingly throughout the world, and the water-based fuel cell, at present in the development stage.

It is the high efficiency of energy conversion in modern water pumps and turbines that has made pumped storage economically attractive as a means of storing excess base output to help meet peak demand. The capital cost of such schemes is high, \$25 to \$35 per kilowatt being typical. An excellent example, which includes a high man-made reservoir, is the Taum Sauk scheme, Missouri, in which enough water can be raised 280 m. above the generating plant, for seven hours' output of the 350-MW power station. Where possible, in the interest of economy, high-level natural lakes are used for pumped-storage schemes. The Ffestiniog scheme, in northern Wales, is of this type. Here the natural reservoir is situated 325 m. above, and only 8 km. distant from, the 500-MW nuclear power station at Trawsfynydd. The four pumps installed to raise the water are rated at 75 MW each, and the total generating capacity of the power station is 320 MW.

Several types of fuel cell have been proposed for the large-scale storage of electrical energy, of which only the hydrogen-

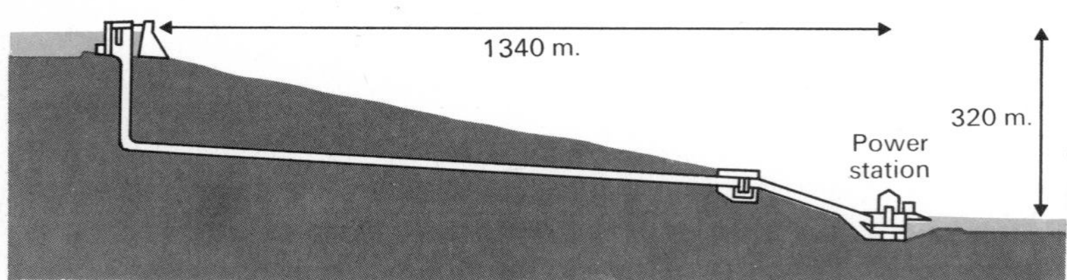

Above: cross section of the Ffestiniog pumped-storage hydroelectric scheme in North Wales. Four pumps, powered by conventional generating plant and rated at 75 MW each, are used for six or seven hours during the night to fill the upper reservoir. The four Francis turbine/generator units (above the pumps in the power station) can be used at maximum output (80 MW each) for four hours the following day. The plant can be used as a standby for extreme peak demand (category C, page 117). Below: a view across the lower reservoir, showing the power station and upper dam.

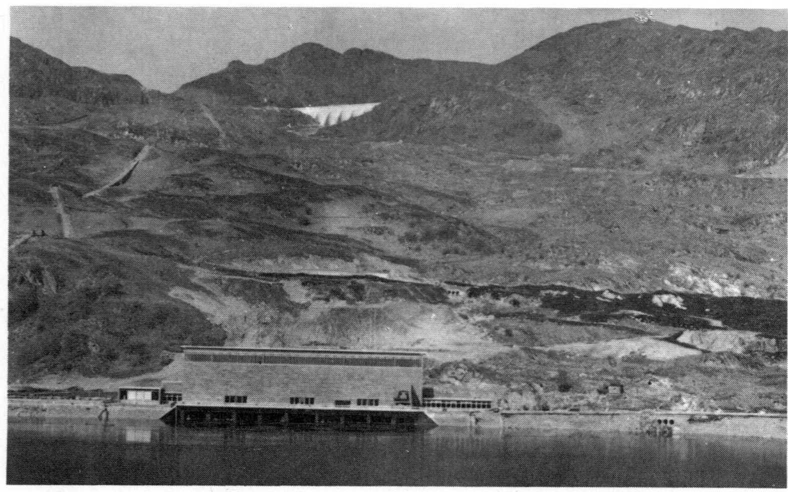

oxygen fuel cell has currently been shown to be commercially practical. The principle is simple: water is electrolyzed, using excess off-peak current; the oxygen and hydrogen liberated are then stored under pressure (about 100 atmospheres is proposed) in large-bore underground cylinders. At times of peak demand the oxygen and hydrogen are reconverted into water in a fuel cell, liberating electricity. To store as much energy as the Ffestiniog pumped-storage reservoir requires the electrolysis of about 425,000 kg. of water, producing 50,000 kg. of hydrogen and 375,000 kg. of oxygen. Accommodation of these quantities of gases at 100 atmospheres would require 300 m. of 6-m-diameter mild-steel underground cylinder for the hydrogen and 150 m. for the oxygen. This is a comparatively simple installation that would cost only about \$2¾ million, far less than a comparable reservoir for pumped storage. Fuel cells for the conversion process could vary in design but present knowledge suggests the use of porous nickel electrodes operating in an aqueous solution of potassium hydroxide under 40 atmospheres pressure, at a temperature of about 200°C. Working at an overall efficiency of about 50 per cent, a continuous power output of about 2000 W/m^2 of electrode could be achieved in a cell delivering 0.85 volts. Suitably designed on the basis of this unit a fuel cell plant with an output of 1200 megawatt hours (MWh)—that of Ffestiniog—is technically possible. The total cost of such a plant would work out in the region of \$100 per kilowatt. At first sight this would appear to make the system's commercial viability highly doubtful. However, any

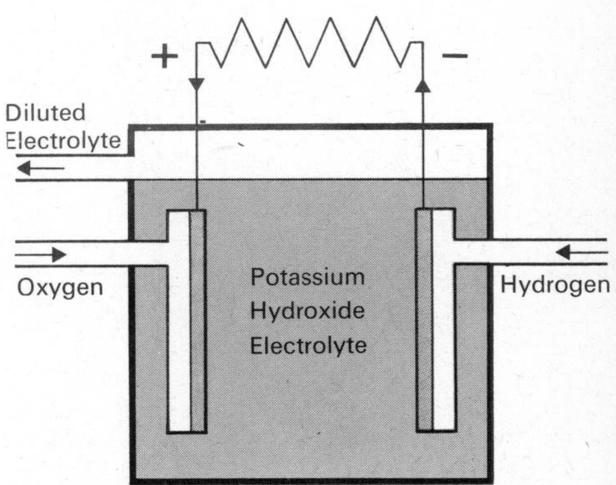

Fuel cells are simple devices that continuously convert chemical energy into electrical energy. Shown is a low-temperature, low-pressure, hydrogen-oxygen unit containing an electrolyte of 30% potassium hydroxide solution. Hydrogen and oxygen gas pass through the porous wall of the hollow electrodes (several interleaved) and react to form water and electrons, which flow as current. Hydroelectricity could be used to electrolyze water into hydrogen and oxygen gas, which could be reconverted into electricity in a large-scale version of this cell.

research that results in lowering the capital cost of fuel cell construction might quickly turn the scales in favor of the electrolytic fuel cell.

Economics of Power Production

No one can afford to spend millions of dollars on a project to produce power if the cost of producing that power is uncompetitive. Though the production of electricity almost always seems to fall short of demand, there is a limit to the price even industry will pay.

On the face of it one would expect hydroelectric power to be relatively cheaper than alternative sources, since there is no fuel to pay for. In practice this is not necessarily so. Accountants do not always agree on the method of calculating the true cost of operating a large plant. Figures can be juggled with in various ways. The cost of producing hydroelectric power may be divided into three elements: interest on and repayment of the capital cost of the plant and associated civil engineering; renewal expenses in respect of wear and tear; direct operating expenses. It may be presumed that the capital required to carry out any large project of this nature, involving the building of a dam, aqueducts or water tunnels, a power station, and facilities to convey the power produced to the appropriate center of consumption (often many kilometers away) is borrowed money. And since very large sums are likely to be involved we can assume that the loans are long-term and that the interest payable is low. In fact where the government participates 5 per cent is a likely interest on a loan repayable in 80 years. Renewal expenses, financed by a depreciation fund, may be relatively large. A power complex looks permanent enough at the time of the opening ceremony, but not even a dam will last for ever. Typical lives of the various components are:

Dams and major aqueducts	80–100 years
Buildings	40–50 years
Water control gear	30–40 years
Generating plant and transmission lines	25–35 years
Switchgear and transformers	20–30 years

When allocating funds for possible future renewals one uncomfortable fact emerges. The value of money is forever falling, and if we base our renewal fund on the original cost of the various components, our children will probably find it quite impossible to rebuild or replace with the same sum when renewal can no longer be postponed. This means that either the electricity consumer must pay two, three, or even four times today's production price toward the cost of renewal by his children, or he must bequeath to them the problem of finding additional funds when the occasion arises. One might almost say that this is a problem of ethics. Accountants disagree; they have their own theories. Certainly future costs can affect the price of hydroelectric power today.

Direct operating costs need no elaboration; they include staff salaries, maintenance and repairs, insurance, and office expenses. In practice the total annual cost of running a major hydroelectric plant is found to vary from about $10\frac{1}{2}$ to 12 per cent of the capital involved. What is particularly interesting is the fact that almost half of this cost is interest on the original loan. However violently the economy may inflate and currency depreciate, the account book is satisfied with a constant interest payment such that, while renewal costs rise, the cost of hydroelectric power can fall with the passing years without the undertaking being out of pocket. This is in sharp contrast to the cost of power produced from conventional fuels, where fuel cost is a major component of power cost, and, because fuel costs are always rising, so must the cost of the power produced.

The cost of hydroelectric power can be further, sometimes dramatically, influenced by what at first sight appear to be unrelated factors. Many great dams, for example, are designed not only as a provision for water storage and a working head for power production, but as an integral part of an irrigation scheme. The water diverted into canals after passing through the turbines may bring in a revenue greater than the cost of its distribution. Even where the diverted water is distributed at cost, the area will produce more crops, become richer, and pay higher taxes. If the power authority is the government they might consider a measure of subsidy justifiable where the price of power production would otherwise work out too high to attract sufficient consumers in the early years of a project. A more tangible, yet equally indirect and apparently unrelated, income at a hydroelectric plant may be found in the collection of tolls for the use of a roadway built along the rim of a great dam. Such a roadway might well shorten a route across a valley by many kilometers, saving transport operators many liters of gasoline. By paying the toll they might be saving themselves expense. Yet the hydroelectric authority receives an income and no one makes a loss.

There would be little point in trying to pin down the cost of hydroelectric power more precisely. The principles should now be clear. The actual cost will vary widely in relation to the many factors involved. And even if the cost in a particular case may be high in relation to the cost of conventional or nuclear power stations in the area, the facility of immediately being able to fill those sometimes unpredictable peaks in the electrical demand curve may be worth more to the undertaking than the additional cost of producing that power. The accountant may write his figures here in red; the managing director knows that without doing this he cannot keep his customers satisfied and thereby keep the very much larger account for the steady output in the blue. Sometimes, indeed, the boot may be on the other foot. The Aswan High Dam has been built because Egypt cannot continue to grow without the water it impounds. The power produced is a bonus. Who is to say what it costs?

The Industrial Potential of Hydroelectric Power

We have seen how interest on capital is a major component in the cost of hydroelectric power. The prime source of the energy to be converted costs nothing and therefore the nearer a hydroelectric plant can run to maximum output (in other words, the higher the load factor it can achieve), the lower the cost of the power produced. This is true of other forms of power production, but applies especially to power cost of the hydroelectric station. Where power is cheap, or potentially cheap, industry must thrive. Where potential hydroelectric energy greatly exceeds demand, the growth of large-scale power-consuming industry may substantially lower the cost of producing the power.

One industry that consumes huge quantities of power is the aluminum-producing industry, which is today in a phase of rapid growth and shows no signs of abatement. Indeed the current and foreseeable demand for this metal is such that, where a supply of inexpensive power is assured, its production cannot be other than profitable. Consequently, wherever the potential of hydroelectric power production is great and existing electricity demand low (a situation that, in normal circumstances, would inhibit the construction of any large and costly power plant), it may well be that the founding of an aluminum-smelting industry can be so encouraged by the offer of low-cost electrical power that the growth of that industry makes the production of hydroelectric power economic. The area then reaps a double benefit. Not only does it acquire a source of cheap power for all other purposes, but it develops economically by the introduction of local industry on a relatively large scale. All this because the presence of a high head source of water has been economically exploited by engineering.

Again, an area may be potentially fertile, but too dry for economic crop production. The diversion of water may bring life to the land; but soon the fertility becomes depleted. Then fertilizer is required and, for its economic production, an abundant source of cheap power is also necessary. The water that is now impounded for diversion to the fields is harnessed on its journey and made to yield its potential energy for the production of electricity. In this instance it is the development and continued prosperity of agriculture that has justified the capital expenditure for a dam and a hydroelectric power station. When the irrigation, power, and fertilizer factory complex is completed, a formerly poor and arid area may be transformed into a rich community. The fertilizer replaces the salts that are leached from the soil in irrigation, and agriculture can flourish. The cheap electricity encourages the growth of other industries and with them a new population. Thus, a hydroelectric power station may form the nucleus of a wealthy settlement with a balanced agricultural-industrial economy.

Power from the Tides

The latent energy of the constantly moving tides has fascinated inventive man since earliest days. In theory it should be possible to harness the wasted tidal energy everywhere, even where the tidal range is low. In practice any power we can wrest from tidal action proves uneconomic in the state of current technology, where the tidal range averages less than 10 m. In addition, there must be substantial estuaries or other coastal basins that can conveniently be dammed. Sites fulfilling both these conditions are to be found in barely 5 per cent of the world's coastlines. Also, they are widely scattered, many of them situated far from centers of population and industry. However, four of the best potential sites are near enough to major electricity demand areas to have stimulated serious consideration of development. These are at Passamaquoddy Bay where the US and Canadian east coasts meet, the Severn estuary on the west coast of England, the land-locked White Sea in the northwest corner of Russia, and at several locations along the western reaches of the north coast of France. The Passamaquoddy project, first proposed in 1920 and finally given the green light by President Kennedy in 1963, has been held up by the US Congress not having found the time (or perhaps the inclination) to vote the necessary funds. The Severn estuary scheme, also first considered in 1920 and re-

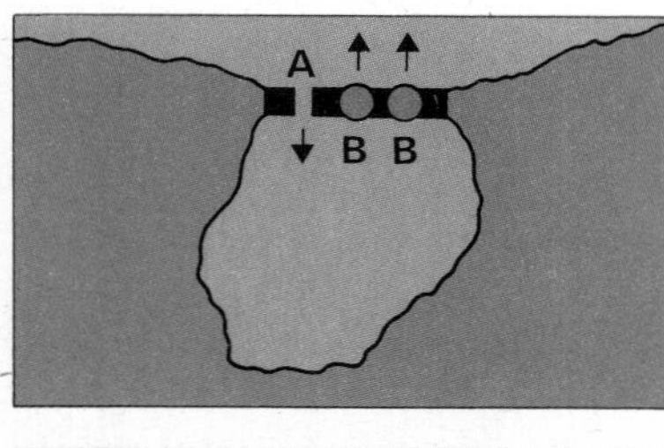

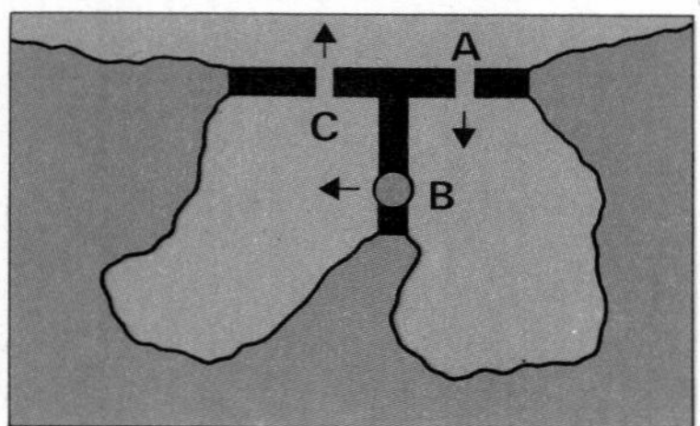

Top left: a single-basin tidal power system. At high tide, seawater flows into the basin and the sluice gates (A) are closed. At low tide, the water is allowed to flow through the turbines (B) back into the sea. Bottom left: a twin-basin tidal power system. At high tide, gates (A) are open and gates (C) are closed. As the tide turns gates (A) are closed and water passes through the turbines (B) to the left-hand basin, which contains water at low-tide level. As this basin fills up, gates (C) are opened and a constant flow is maintained through the turbines. Right: aerial view of the completed Rance barrage, France. From left to right: navigation lock; generating station; fixed dyke; sluice gates.

viewed by the British government several times since, has been indefinitely shelved in favor of nuclear power development. At the White Sea site, Soviet engineers have so far built only a pilot plant for experiment. The French, on the other hand, pushed their first project through to completion in 1966, and today possess the world's first and only commercial tidal power station, on the Rance estuary between the resorts of Saint-Malo and Dinard.

In its simplest form a tidal power plant consists of a low dam across the mouth of a tidal basin—a *single-basin* system. Sluice gates are incorporated at one point, low-head power-generating plant at another. The tide is allowed to flow naturally, via the sluices, into the basin. At high tide the gates are closed and as soon as the sea level has dropped sufficiently to create a usable head of water in the basin (three meters is about the minimum) the trapped water is released via the generators. This basic form of tidal power station has a major disadvantage. Not only is power supply intermittent, but the timing of the output is entirely dependent on the ebb and flow of the tide. Such a plant can therefore neither provide a steady base output nor possess the ability to meet peak load requirements as and when they arise. Even total output, confined to about one third of the full tidal cycle, is too low to be economic. The capital cost is considerable.

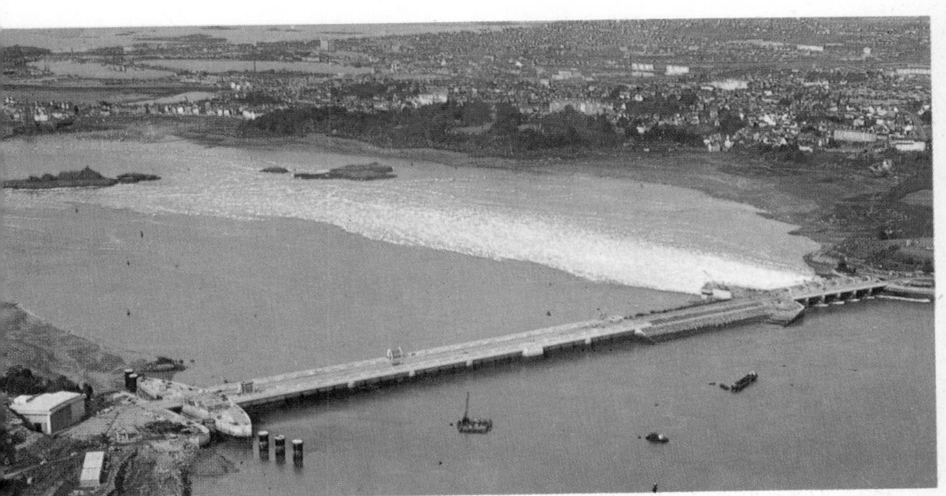

An improved output-to-time ratio can be achieved in several ways. The first is to generate during the flow as well as the ebb of the tide by using turbines designed to operate in either direction. This expedient makes it possible to obtain a useful power conversion factor for about 54 per cent of the tidal cycle. If the turbo-alternators can be designed to pump efficiently as well as to generate electricity, a further improvement in output can be obtained by speeding up the time taken naturally for the changing water levels to reach the minimum working head. While this appears suspiciously like robbing Peter to pay Paul, in practice a power gain of about 1.8 can be achieved by properly timed pumping. Now, if we can design a turbogenerator that not only generates but pumps efficiently in either direction, the total gain in efficiency must clearly be greater than either arrangement alone. An entirely different approach to the problem is represented by the *twin-basin* system (the Passamaquoddy project is, in fact, a multiple basin scheme—a sophisticated variation of the twin-basin principle). This provides a

Cross section of the Rance tidal power barrage, France. Shown is one of 24 bulb turbines, each containing a turbo-alternator of 10-MW capacity. The sluice gates (A) are opened when the difference in water levels between the sea and the reservoir is sufficient for operation of the turbines. Water flows through radial guide-vanes, which are adjusted to maintain maximum turbine efficiency at different heads.

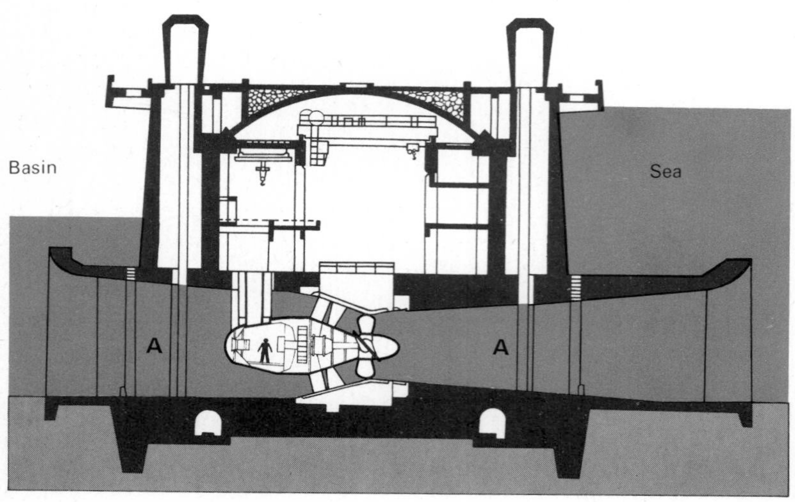

constant working head between two separate basins, and thus makes the timing of power output independent of the times of rise and fall of the tide.

The Rance power station is a single-basin scheme operating in an estuary that provides an average spring tide range of 10.9 m., the equinoctial maximum touching 13.5 m. with a top flood tide flow of about 18,000 m^3/sec. The engineering works are made up of four elements. To the west is a navigation lock, used mainly for fishing and tourist boat traffic; east of this is the 370-m-long power station proper, in which 24 low-head bulb generators are installed within a hollow concrete dam wall; next is a 178-m. rockfill embankment dam, linking the power station to a small island in the estuary. Between the island and the east bank is a 150-m. control barrage with six vertical sluice gates. A two-way highway passes over the top of the engineering works, shortening the road distance from Saint-Malo to Dinard by about 30 km. and, by toll collection, contributing significantly to the revenue of the power station.

The bulb generators used in this scheme are of the very latest design. They have a 10-MW maximum output and are designed both to generate and to pump efficiently in either direction (see opposite). A major problem here was that of seawater corrosion. Extensive research preceded the decision to construct the generator runner blades of either of two alloys, an aluminum bronze, or a high-chrome-content stainless steel with nickel molybdenum. Both materials have in fact been used, providing Electricité de France, the owners, with the opportunity to continue long-term corrosion research under operating conditions. French engineers have therefore become the first to put into service a full-scale tidal electric power station, with a capacity of 240 MW and an estimated net annual output of 544,000 MWh. It has cost about $90 million. So pleased are the French that already they are working out the details for a much larger project designed to impound 400 km^2 of the sea in the Mont-Saint-Michel Bay east of Saint-Malo, not very far from the Rance.

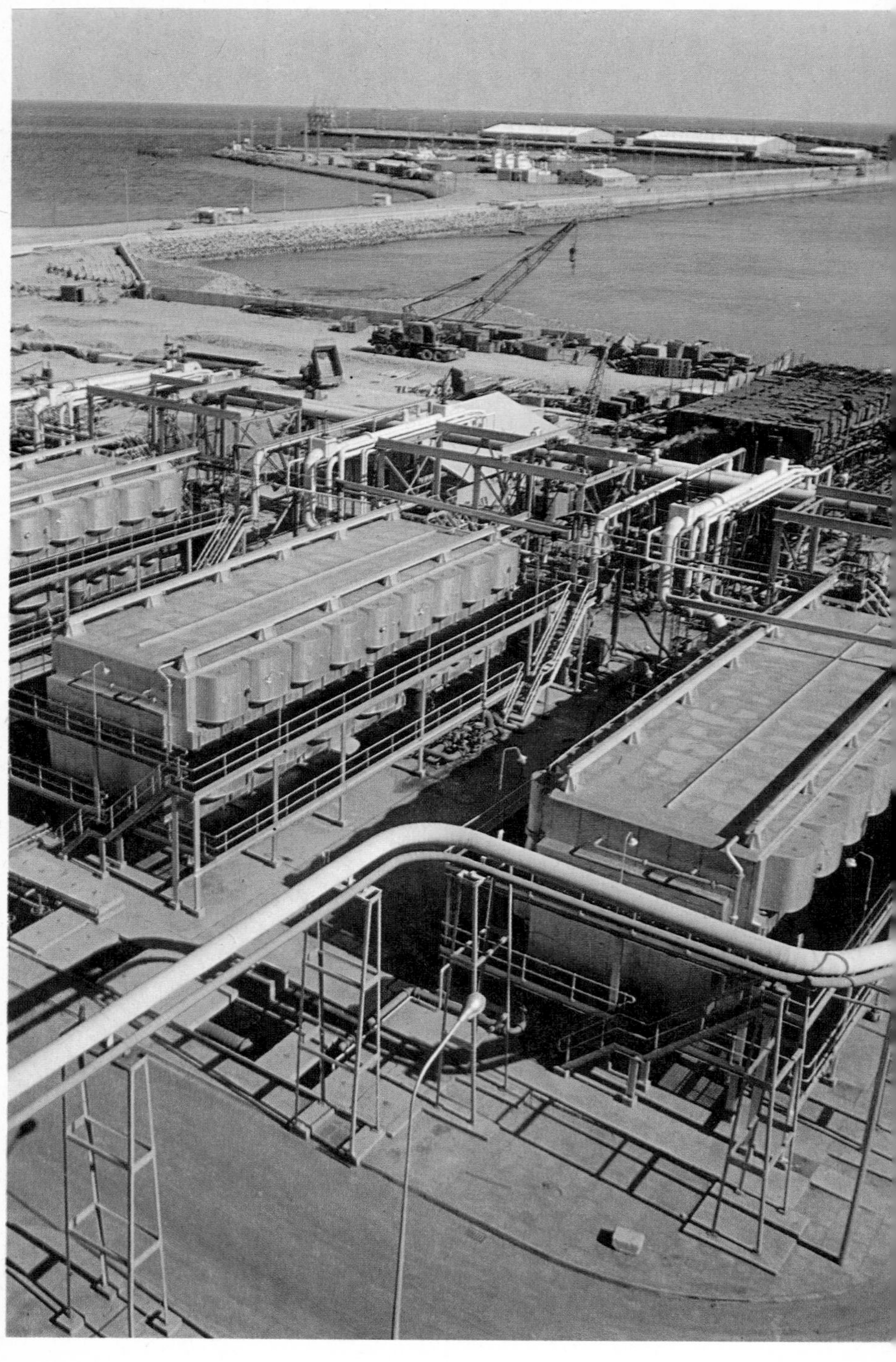

6 Desalination

"Water, water everywhere, nor any drop to drink." No one can sum up more concisely than the Ancient Mariner man's ultimate problem in the quest for water. The water of the oceans laps mockingly at his feet—all 1.6 million Tm^3 of it—but he cannot use it because of the salt it contains. The fact that some 50 of the known elements are represented in the sea's dissolved salts is of no direct concern to us here; nor even that sodium, magnesium, and potassium are present in large enough quantities to warrant their extraction commercially. But we are very much concerned with what the sea's average $3\frac{1}{2}$ per cent salt concentration means in terms of its removal. Calculation reveals that if the oceans were all evaporated and the salts spread evenly over the earth's surface, the resulting layer would be 65 m. thick. In terms of weight this means that one cubic kilometer of seawater contains about 40 million metric tons of salts—in other words, 1 m^3 contains roughly 40 kg.

Desalination of seawater provides a possible solution to local water shortage problems. In Kuwait, the government has commissioned five desalination plants (of the multistage flash-distillation type) to provide the capital city with 22,500 m^3 of fresh water a day.

Of course the sea is not the only source of salt water that man can desalinate. All water, even so-called fresh water, contains some salt. Indeed, drinking water with a salt content of 0.05 per cent or less is rated acceptable for municipal supply by the United States health authorities, and this concentration is in fact virtually unnoticeable. Between the two natural extremes of seawater and "sweet" water lies what is called *brackish* water, containing a substantially lower concentration of salts than the sea, but considerably more than the minimum acceptable in drinking water. Brackish groundwater is the source of the saline springs, famous for their curative properties, that are not uncommon in many parts of the world. Much of the world's natural brackish water exists in the drier latitudes, especially in the Middle East. It is sometimes found in lakes, but more commonly underground. Typical brackish water in the water-short regions of the Middle East has a salt content of about 0.5 per cent, and there is much of it to be had. So here is a source of water, apart from the sea, that could be desalted for human consumption; and it has the virtue of existing inland.

Before 1945 the only desalination plant in regular use was that installed in large ocean-going passenger ships. But water shortages have prompted a rapidly growing research and development effort, especially in the United States, Great Britain, Israel, and Russia. The majority of desalination plants around the world that are working as a commercial proposition are of modest size, producing about 22,500 m^3/day. The total production of desalinated water in Kuwait of 87,600 m^3/day at the end of 1966 represents the total produced by several separate plants. Really large-capacity plants are still at the design stage. In the United States the Office of Saline Water, Washington, DC, is financing a massive research program, and several experimental plants have been built. One of these, a long-tube vertical distillation plant at Freeport, Texas, was originally designed to produce 3750 m^3/day, but subsequently new stages have been added to increase production (see page 140). The most ambitious American project is that of a combined nuclear-power and desalination plant in southern California designed to deliver 568,000 m^3/day (see page 136).

The relative size of such a plant can be appreciated when one considers that the total installed capacity of desalination plants around the world at the end of 1966 was 200,000 m^3/day. Israel is currently considering construction of a plant that will deliver 455,000 m^3/day, and Soviet Russia is planning a plant of 125,000 m^3/day capacity, to be sited at Shevchenko on the Caspian Sea. These projected plants are, however, unrepresentative of the needs and resources of most countries. The United Kingdom has pioneered and dominated the field of small units for specific local requirements—as in Kuwait, where 60 per cent of installed plant has been built by British firms.

A few of the early desalination plants used fuel oil as their heat source, but the trend has been toward making use of "free" energy from integrated power stations. Several existing plants use solar energy, and the exhaust steam of nuclear power stations is being increasingly utilized in the newer flash-distillation units. This will apply to the Los Angeles plant, as well as to those scheduled for early construction in Israel and Russia. Some smaller plants use other "free" sources of energy, notably one on Long Island, New York, that utilizes heat from burning refuse, and one in Peru where the waste heat from a copper-smelting factory is used.

Desalination by Distillation

It is easy to drop a teaspoonful of salt into a tumbler of water; but not so easy to take it out again, leaving the water pure. Distillation is obviously one possible method, but whether water can be distilled cheaply enough for general use is quite another matter. In practice four different methods of distillation have been developed. One of these, known as *multistage flash distillation* (MSF for short), is used in almost all existing plants. This process depends on the vapor that flashes off from hot water when the pressure is reduced. Boiling does not occur.

As fresh water is separated from seawater, brine is formed. It is this that circulates through much of the MSF plant, and from which most fresh water is obtained. The complete process can be subdivided into two main sections. In the more productive of these, brine is pumped under pressure into condenser coils at the top of serially arranged cylindrical tanks called *flash chambers*. The outflow of one condenser becomes the inflow of the next and so on. The brine leaving the coil of the last chamber enters a steam-fed heat exchanger (essentially another coil in a steam jacket), where its temperature is raised to 80°C. This is purposely kept below boiling point for reasons that will be explained later. The hot liquid then passes back into the flash chambers, but this time as a free-running flow across the base of each tank and in the opposite direction to that flowing in the condensers. Because in each sealed tank the air is at reduced pressure, water vapor flashes off the surface of the brine and condenses on the cool surfaces of the coil. Troughs immediately below the condensers collect and convey the fresh water to the main outflow system. The important consideration is that as the brine temperature falls in each succeeding tank (the latent heat of evaporation is extracted from it), a correspondingly lower pressure must be maintained for flashing-off to occur.

A counter-current heat exchange system is also in operation as the heat lost by the "free" brine warms the piped brine on its way to the main heat exchanger. The now cooler (60°C) and more concentrated salt solution enters the base of another flash chamber; the first of a series comprising the next main section of the plant. Here the condenser coils contain raw seawater, and at a greatly reduced pressure (commensurate with the now

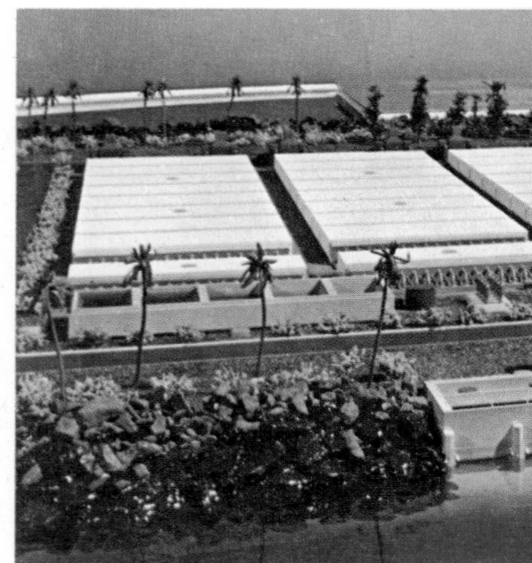

A model of the proposed combined nuclear-power station and desalination plant to be built on a man-made island about 40 km. south of Los Angeles. The project, directed by the Office of Saline Water and at a total estimated cost of $500 million, incorporates two large conventional light-water nuclear reactors providing energy for generating plant of 1800 MW output, and three multistage flash distillation plants of 568,000 m³/day combined capacity. The estimated date of completion is 1972.

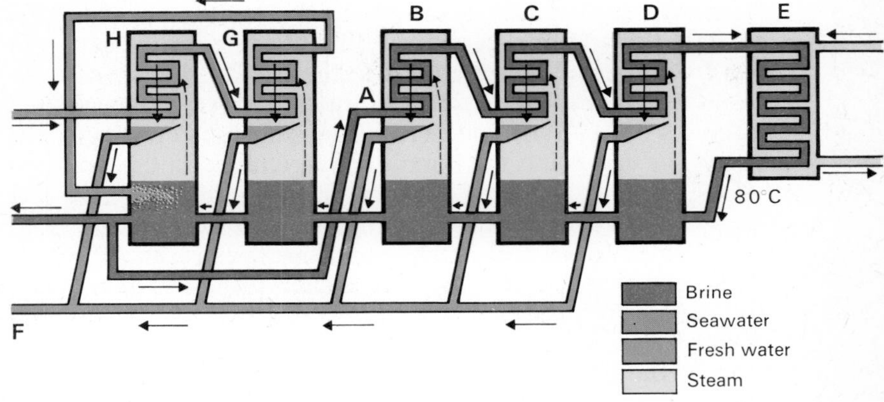

The multistage flash-distillation process. Brine at (A) passes under pressure in the condenser coils of flash chambers (B), (C), and (D), to heat exchanger (E), and, as it flows in the reverse direction, water vapor flashes off and is condensed on the cooler brine-filled coils above. The condensate forms part of the freshwater outflow at (F). The brine, now at 60°C, passes into flash chambers (G) and (H), which contain condenser coils fed with raw seawater. This is recycled into the concentrated brine of the last flash chamber and the resultant liquid is partly run off as waste and partly recycled to (A). From right to left the flash chambers operate at a progressively reduced temperature and pressure.

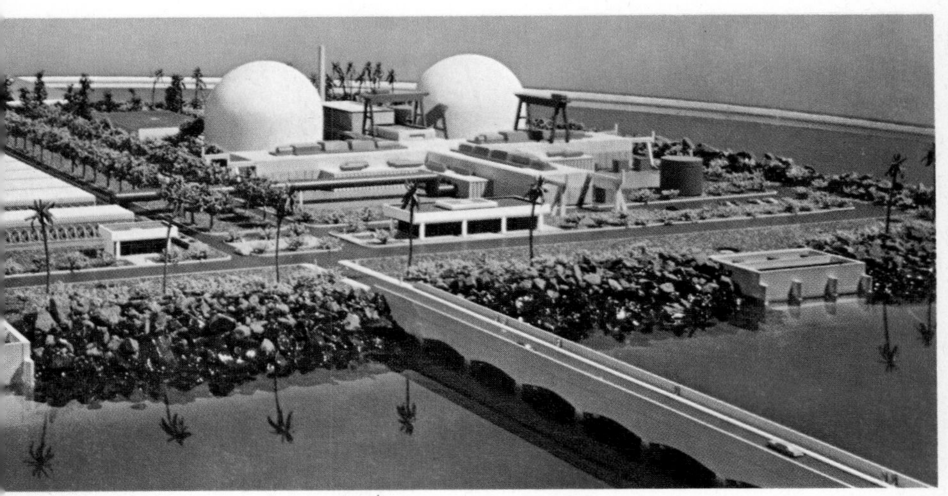

lowered temperature) flash distillation occurs as before. The seawater (flowing in the opposite direction from the brine) is piped from the condenser coils into the base of the last distillation tank, where it adds to and dilutes the very concentrated outflowing brine. Some of the resulting solution (7 per cent salt) is run off as waste and the remainder is pumped under pressure to the condenser coils of the first flash chamber series. The complete cycle thus requires input of steam and seawater, from which brine waste and fresh water are produced. Part recycling of the brine results in a higher ratio of fresh water produced per unit of feed steam, lowering the cost of the final fresh water produced (see page 137).

One of the problems of distillation is the formation of scale in the hot brine circulating system. Calcium carbonate and magnesium hydroxide scale were formerly controlled by dosing with a proprietary chemical effective up to a temperature of 85°C, which explains why the brine is not heated above 80°C, although higher temperatures would in theory result in improved performance at reduced capital expense. Research has been actively seeking other methods of scale control. One method has been devised to inhibit calcium carbonate ($CaCO_3$) and magnesium hydroxide ($Mg[OH]_2$) scale formation up to 120°C, when calcium sulfate scaling sets in. Seeding and ion exchange processes are also under development for the control of sulfate scaling and it is likely that future plant will be designed to operate at temperatures up to 150°C or even 175°C, with higher pressures to prevent the brine from boiling. This should substantially reduce the cost of fresh water produced, though it would not be possible in dual-purpose plants where exhaust steam from turbines is used as a cheap source of heat, and where the temperature of this feed steam is relatively low. An interesting use of the multistage flash-distillation process is to be found in a recent British design for a desalination ship, intended to supply fresh water to island communities in times of emergency. This 55-m-long ship, having a displacement of 1300 metric tons, would desalinate 100 m^3 of seawater a day.

Where high-temperature steam is available as the heat source, distillation by boiling can be achieved economically by using a series of evaporators. One such system is *multiple-effect long-tube vertical distillation* (LTV). Raw seawater is fed into the top of the first of a series of evaporators and falls as a film down the inside of long vertical tubes. A steam jacket surrounding these causes the water to boil on its downward journey, the resulting hot water vapor is led away, and brine collects in the base of the unit. The high-temperature feed steam condenses to fresh water and joins the main outflow. In the next and subsequent evaporators the water vapor from the previous unit is used as the jacket heat source and, as it condenses, becomes part of the fresh water product. Each evaporator operates at a slightly lower temperature than the preceding one (see diagram on page 140).

In contrast to this the *vapor compression distillation* plant operates mainly on a mechanical rather than a heat energy source. Raw seawater (plus recycled brine) is pumped into the base of a vertical evaporator and surrounds the lower part of several vertical tubes, the open ends of which project into a steam-filled space above. Halfway up the unit, steam is introduced under pressure below the surface of the seawater, and by evaporation extra steam is produced, some of which travels down the vertical tubes, condensing to fresh water in the cooled lower regions of the tank, and thence to the main outflow system. Some of the steam is drawn off, recompressed, and recycled. After an initial input of steam the plant operates continuously on the mechanical energy of the seawater/brine recycling pump and the steam compressor, both of which can be conveniently driven by electricity (see diagram on page 141).

This process has been much used in small plants, especially on board ship. The only large plant in existence, built at Roswell, New Mexico, and designed to deliver about 3000 m^3 of fresh water daily, has proved disappointing. While in theory this process has a low energy consumption, in practice the high cost of the power used to drive the compressors and the high capital cost of the mechanical element in the plant has resulted in the cost of fresh water produced being too high to warrant commercial development of the process.

On the Greek island of Patmos, dry summers had forced the

government to ship fresh water from the mainland at enormous cost. The local system of supply, comprising five small reservoirs (total capacity 2500 m^3) fed by the water that collected during the short rainy season in a ravine near the only township, had proved inadequate, even when augmented by pumping from a well and by rain guttered from the roof of each house. Because the island is poor and could not afford expensive water, the Technical University of Athens designed a remarkably simple and cheap *solar distillation* plant.

Seawater is pumped to a feed reservoir from which it flows by

Left: the multiple-effect long-tube vertical distillation process. Seawater entering at (A) boils as it passes down the tubes (B), and the resulting steam is used as the heat source for the next unit. Steam from the previous unit (or high-temperature feed steam, if this unit is the first of the series) enters at (C) and condenses to fresh water. This joins the main outflow at (D). Right: the experimental LTV plant at Freeport, Texas, of 3750 m^3/day capacity. Extra stages have been built to increase this capacity, and the plant has been found to operate as economically as existing types of flash distillation. It cannot, however, compete in costs with plant using "free" low-temperature steam.

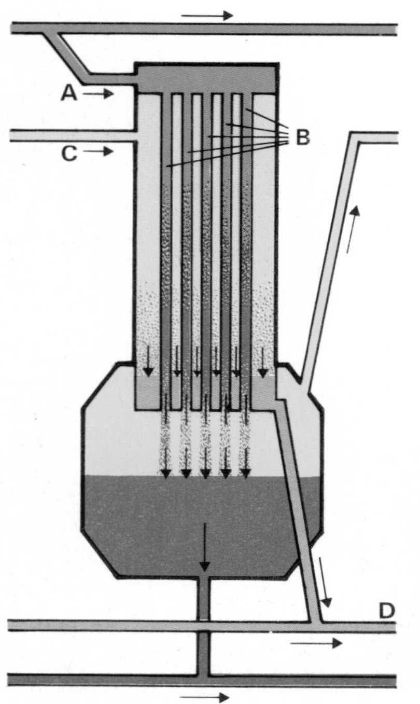

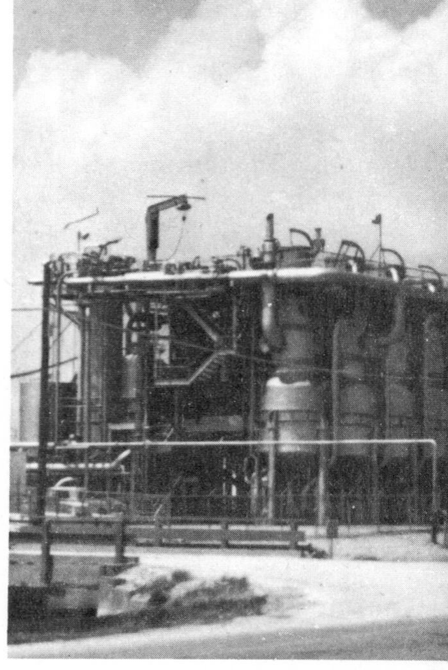

gravity, when required, into a large shallow basin divided into long narrow sections. Separating these channels are concrete strips, which provide access for maintenance. The interior surface of the entire basin is lined with butyl rubber sheet. Above each water-filled section is a double sloping glass roof supported by a light aluminum structure. Heat from the sun passes through the glass, causing evaporation from the seawater surface. The vapor condenses on the inside of the glass and runs down to channels at the edges of the sealed unit, along which it travels to the freshwater storage reservoir. The salt

Left: the vapor compression distillation process. Seawater and recycled brine are circulated by pump (E) around the condenser tubes (F). Compressor (G) forces steam under pressure into the salt water, evaporating it and so supplying more steam to the compressor. Some steam condenses in the vertical tubes and forms the freshwater output at (H). Right: the experimental vapor compression plant at Roswell, New Mexico. Designed to deliver 3000 m³/day, this plant has shown that, due to high energy and equipment costs per unit output, the process is not yet commercially economical.

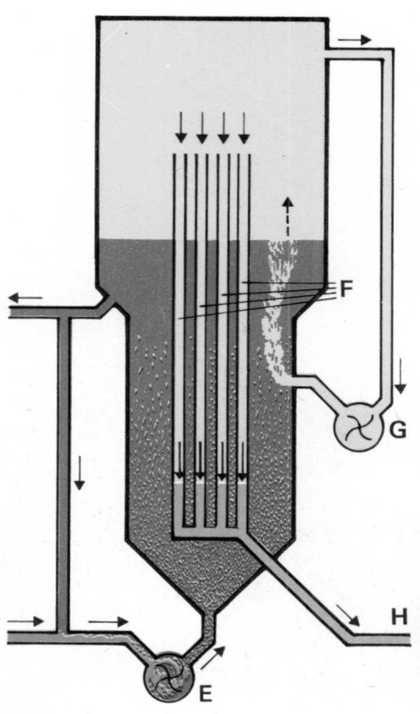

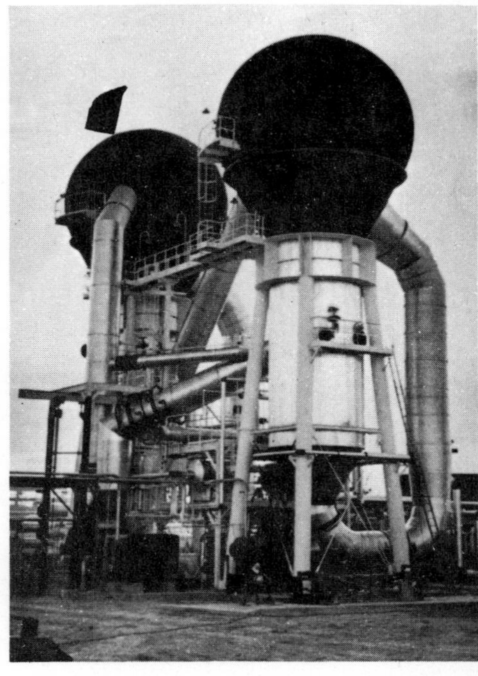

concentration in the basin sections grows steadily stronger, and once every two days the resulting brine is run off to the sea, being then replaced by more seawater. Experience has shown that the 48-hour cycle avoids the formation of scale. As the sun does not shine every day, the designers incorporated a second water channel in the concrete strips. These are fed from the upper surface of the glass panels, and from the concrete itself, when it rains (see diagram on this page).

The output of distilled water from the Patmos solar still averages three liters per square meter of water surface per day. With a total evaporation area of about 9000 m^2 the total yield is about 27 m^3 of fresh water daily. The average annual rainfall of 60 cm. almost exactly doubles this output. Only 54 m^3 of water a day sounds insignificant after the figures we have been

Principle of a solar still. Evaporation occurs at the surface of the seawater (A); vapor condenses on the inside of the sloping glass panels (B) and runs down into the inside collecting channels (C). Rainwater (D) runs down the outside of the glass panels and from the concrete access strip (E) and collects in the outside channels (F). After a week enough heat is concentrated to provide continuous day and night distillation.

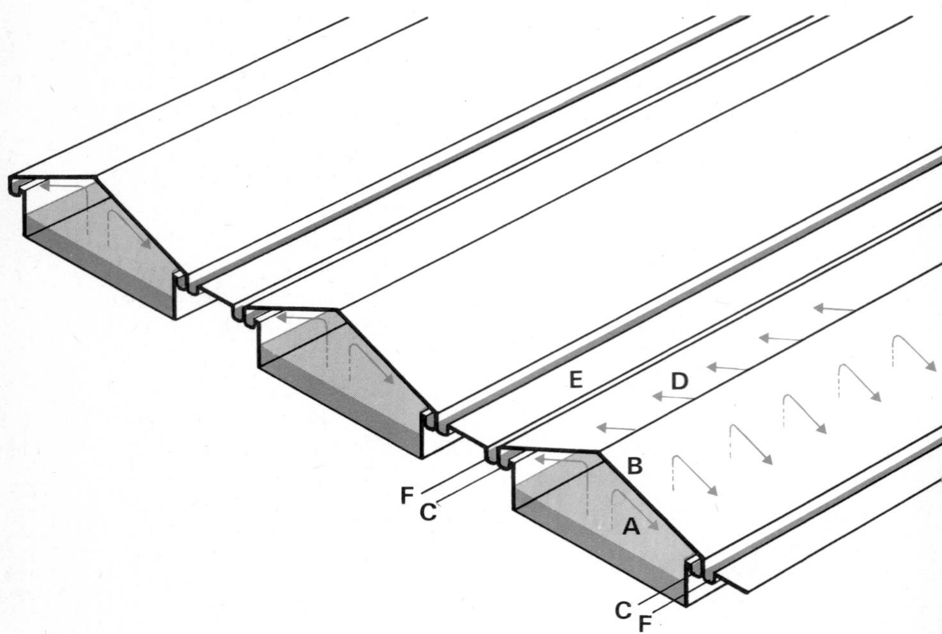

quoting in this book. But with an island population of only 2000 it serves Patmos well, providing every man and woman with an additional 27 liters of fresh water each day, almost free. The only running costs are those of pumping seawater to the feed reservoir, and of general maintenance, which includes cleaning the glass panels.

Electrodialysis

In the Orange Free State, South Africa, there is a desalination plant designed to treat 15,000 m^3 of brackish water daily, by a process in which distillation plays no part. It is an electrochemical process called *electrodialysis*, in which ion transfer separates salt from water. The principle is simple. Salts in solution are ionized, the ions carrying either a positive or a negative charge: e.g. salt (NaCl) becomes, in solution, a mixture of Na(+) and Cl(−) ions. When electrodes, connected to a suitable direct current supply, are immersed in a salt solution (e.g. seawater), current will flow, carried by the ions. The ions with a positive charge are attracted toward the negative *cathode* and are called *cations*. Negatively charged *anions* flow toward the positive *anode*. This is the working principle of *electrolysis*. In electrodialysis, filters or membranes, selectively impervious to cations or anions, are placed alternately between the electrodes. Cation filters permit the flow of anions but act as a barrier to positively charged cations. Conversely, anions are held back by the anion filter while cations pass through unchecked. In certain compartments of the tank, ions will collect as their flow is checked by the appropriate filter. Cells of increasing salt concentration thus alternate with cells of salt depletion. Water sufficiently deionized (i.e. desalinated) is extracted from the appropriate compartments (see page 144).

In actual installations the ion-permeable membranes are built into a unit, known as a *stack*, that operates and looks quite like a filter press. The brackish water is pumped through the stack, producing an outlet water that is partially desalted. Brackish waters with a high salinity require three or four stacks arranged in a series in order to obtain a product of drinking-water quality. This system of desalination works very well, provided the current density across a given area of membrane is not too high: above a certain limit the deposition of scale on the membranes may occur, which will prevent efficient operation. Present-day membranes are reasonably cheap, and sufficiently strong to have an expected lifetime of at least four years.

Research and development are continually taking place on all aspects of the process, and research in the membrane field by a Chicago physicist has produced an inorganic membrane that appears to be stronger and more efficient than the present organic types used. This membrane has proved extremely stable at relatively high temperatures, and laboratory tests have demonstrated a greatly improved desalting action. However, these new cation and anion membranes, based on zirconium and thorium hydroxide respectively, are expensive. It remains to be seen whether they will be suitable for commercial development. Since the energy consumed in electrodialysis is a simple function of the quantity of salt transferred from the diluate to the concentrate compartments, it follows that the cost of fresh water produced by the process will vary with the original salt content. This is not so in the case of distillation. In fact electrodialysis has hitherto been developed primarily for the desalting of brackish water of salinity not exceeding one per

Left: the principle of electrodialysis. Cation membranes (red) alternate with anion membranes (green) in a vertical stack between the electrodes. Brackish water pumped in at (A), (B), (C), and (D) leaves as concentrate at (W) and (Y) and as partially deionized (i.e. desalinated) water at (X) and (Z). Three or four stacks are used in series to produce water of the required purity. Right: laying down ion membranes in a commercial stack.

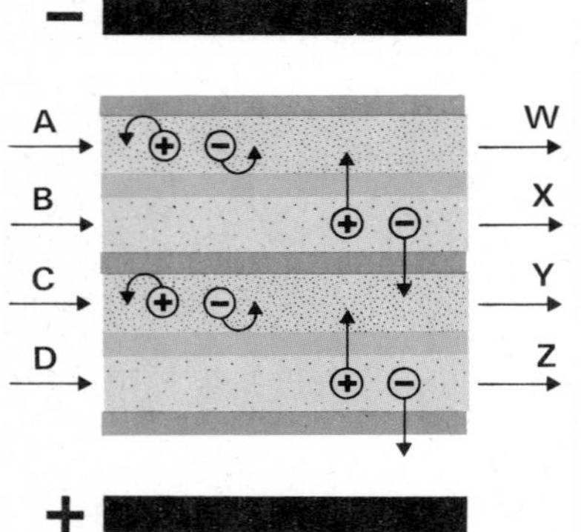

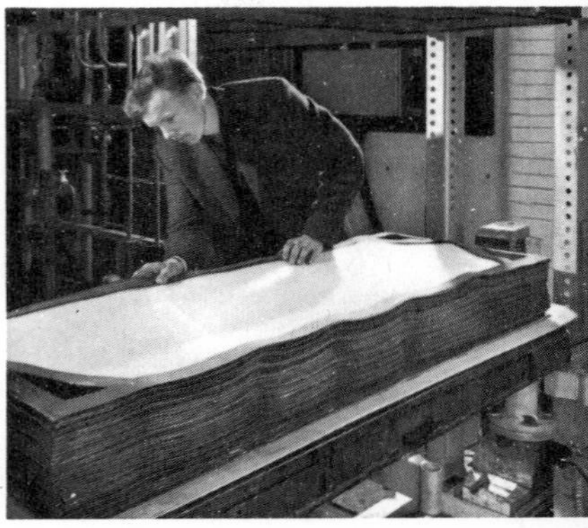

cent, proving uneconomic for water with a higher salt content. At the other end of the range, as the water in the diluate compartments becomes more and more salt free, its resistance to the passage of electricity becomes correspondingly greater and the conversion rate consequently less. Electrodialysis is not therefore used for the reduction of salt content of water below 0.04 per cent. Despite these limitations there are many small electrodialysis plants in commercial use around the world.

The development of electrodialysis has now reached the stage that, between the limits of salt concentration mentioned above, it is the most economically attractive process available at the present time for drinking-water production. The development of new and cheaper membranes may even make it attractive for the production of desalted water for irrigation.

Reverse Osmosis

The properties of a membrane are also made use of in desalination by *reverse osmosis*. When a solution of salt is separated from pure water by a semipermeable membrane that permits the passage of pure water but prevents that of the salt, water will tend to diffuse through the membrane into the salt solution, continuously diluting it. If the salt solution is in an

Left: the principle of reverse osmosis. Brackish water entering at (A) is subjected to a pressure in excess of, and in the opposing direction to, the osmotic pressure operating across the semipermeable membrane (B). Water passes through the membrane and is drawn off at (C). Brine is led away at (D). Right: assembly of an experimental cell using a cellulose acetate semipermeable membrane.

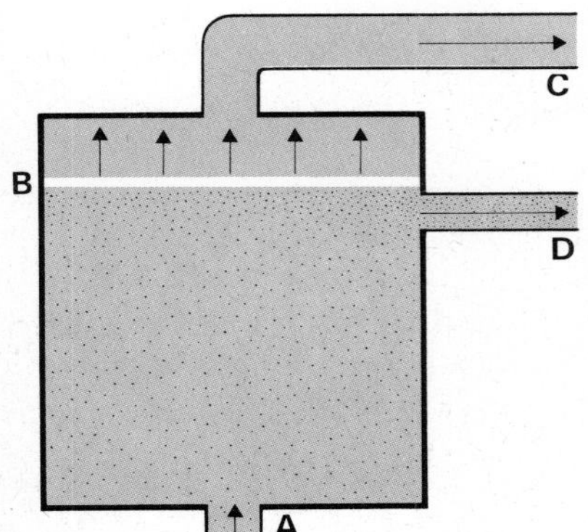

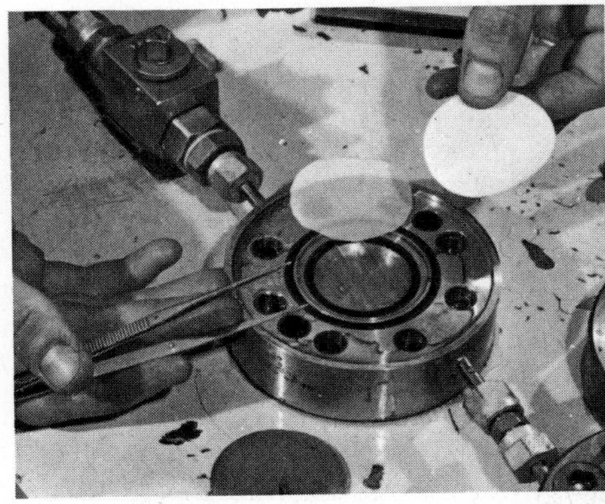

enclosed vessel a pressure will be developed by the inflowing water. This is the well-known natural phenomenon called *osmosis*, and the pressure it can induce in a particular solution is known as the *osmotic pressure* of that solution. In recent years research has been directed to the reverse process, of forcing pure water out of solution by confining it within a semi-permeable membrane and applying a pressure in excess of its natural osmotic pressure. In theory this method should provide an economical means of desalting saline water, as the only energy requirement is that needed to raise and maintain the required pressure. Pure water will then flow naturally through the membrane. By the middle of 1967, researchers in the United States had achieved a reverse osmosis rate of approximately 1 m^3 per square meter of membrane per day from brackish water (0.5 per cent salt), using a working pressure of 500,000 kg/m^2. The desalination of seawater by this process requires much higher pressures for the production of a useful output of fresh water, and pressures as high as one million kg/m^2 have been quoted to produce a freshwater flux of 0.5 m^3 per square meter of membrane daily.

One of the many problems now under investigation is that of providing the currently favored cellulose acetate membranes with the mechanical strength to withstand these high pressures. Possible measures under test for commercial use include placing the membrane against the surface of either disks or tubes of porous fiber glass, or of copper sheet pierced with minute holes. Other experiments have used a spirally wound membrane with sand, or similar inert granular material, as a spacer. The largest experimental reverse osmosis plant built so far is designed to deliver 400 m^3/day—not a great output, but it is confidently anticipated that once a successful membrane suitable for commercial manufacture has been developed, the process will have wide practical application.

Desalination by Freezing

Strangely enough, one of the hottest countries in the world, Israel, uses the phenomenon of ice formation as a basis for a desalination process. This is the *vacuum freeze process*. When salt water is frozen, the crystals that form consist of pure ice, the natural process of crystallization expelling the salt. When this happens, the salt remains in solution as brine on the surface of each pure crystal. The vacuum freeze process for desalination makes use of this fact by freezing salt water, washing the crystals clear of brine, and finally remelting them. However, the ingenious process is more than just that. When atmospheric pressure is reduced, the boiling point of water falls progressively, and by reducing the pressure to 4.6 mm. of mercury absolute (4.6 mm. Hg abs.) the boiling point of water is lowered to 0°C. This, of course, is its freezing point, which is not altered by the change in pressure. At 4.6 mm. Hg abs., therefore, water freezes and boils at the same temperature. This is not as absurd as it first appears, for water's latent heat of vaporization keeps the freezing and boiling phenomena apart in terms of energy input. So if you heat ice at this low pressure it first absorbs the latent heat of fusion, melting to form water at 0°C. After melting, it requires more heat—the latent heat of vaporization—before it will boil, though the temperature of the water vapor formed will still be 0°C. Salt water freezes at a slightly lower temperature than pure water, and to reduce its boiling point to its freezing temperature, as is done in the vacuum freeze process, requires an even lower absolute pressure. The process, in fact, operates at a pressure of 3 mm. Hg abs.

The practical application of vacuum freezing to desalination is carried out in two separate stages. Seawater, at a temperature of about 18°C, is passed through two opposing flow heat exchangers (arranged in parallel), which are fed by freezing brine from the plant and the ice-cold product water respectively. The result of this heat exchange is the lowering of the seawater temperature almost to its freezing point and the warming up of the brine and freshwater output to about 16°C. The cold seawater now enters the lower tank of a hydroconverter (a cylindrical tank divided into upper and lower parts by a peripheral shelf formed centrally into an upwardly directed funnel), in which pressure is reduced to 3 mm. Hg abs. by an exhaust pump. Also entering this tank is freezing brine. As these two flows mix at this low pressure, ice crystals form in the seawater while the brine boils to form water vapor. The salt excluded from the vapor and the ice crystals further concentrates the brine. The brine and ice crystal slurry is pumped to a counterwasher (divided into inner and outer cylindrical tanks), where it passes up the outer tank while fresh water flows down through it, washing the brine from the ice. Pure clean ice crystals reach the top and are forced by a rotating scraper to a chute, which conveys them to the upper tank of the hydroconverter. Here they mix with the water vapor issuing from the central funnel, and pure water at 0°C is formed, the heat of condensation of the vapor providing the heat of fusion of the ice. The fresh water used to wash the ice crystals in the outer counterwasher tank passes, cold and charged with salt, into the inner tank. From here its flow is divided, approximately half forming the brine intake of the lower hydroconverter tank, while the remainder passes through the inflow heat exchanger and then to waste.

The temperature in the counterwasher is controlled by a refrigeration plant supplied with slurry from the hydroconverter. This comparatively small unit pumps freezing brine into the counterwasher when the temperature rises above the working limit (see opposite). This complicated process has been developed by the Israeli government with technical aid from the United States.

An alternative freeze process, the *secondary refrigerant process*, uses butane or a similar liquid hydrocarbon for heat transfer. The butane and feed water pass through a heat exchanger; the transferred heat boils the butane and results in freezing of the water in the brine. The ice crystals are then washed to remove brine, separated, and finally remelted by heat exchange with the butane vapor, which has previously been compressed. There are indications that the secondary refrigerant process is more reliable in operation than the vacuum freeze process.

Still more methods of desalination are under active research today, notably ion exchange systems involving chemical reactions (see Chapter 7), and further freezing techniques. Some success has been reported but none has been developed, at the time of writing, beyond the laboratory stage.

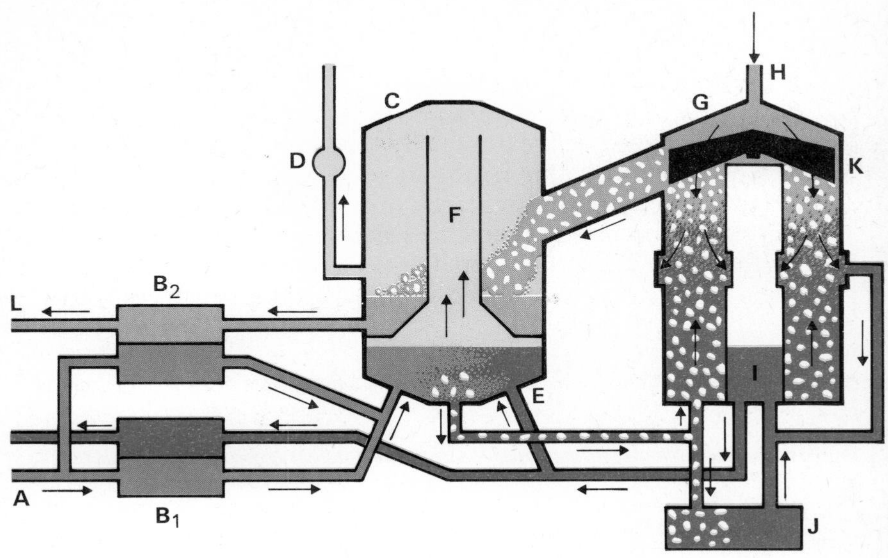

The vacuum freeze desalination process. Above: seawater (18°C) enters at (A), passing through heat exchangers (B_1 and B_2) to the base of the hydroconverter (C). At a pressure of 3 mm. mercury absolute, maintained by exhaust pump (D), the seawater mixes with freezing brine entering at (E). The brine boils, and ice crystals form in the seawater. The water vapor passes up the central funnel (F) and the ice/brine slurry passes to the base of the counterwasher (G): Pure water entering at (H) washes the salt from the ice crystals, and the resulting brine passes into the central counterwasher tank (I). Some of this is recycled to the hydroconverter, and some via heat exchanger (B_1) to waste. The refrigeration plant (J) maintains the working temperature of the counterwasher. Clean ice crystals at the top of the counterwasher are conveyed by the rotating scraper (K) to the upper portion of the hydroconverter. Here the heat of condensation of the vapor provides the heat of fusion of the ice, and pure water at 0°C is formed. This passes through heat exchanger (B_2) and leaves the plant at (L). Below: the vacuum freeze desalination plant at Elath, Israel.

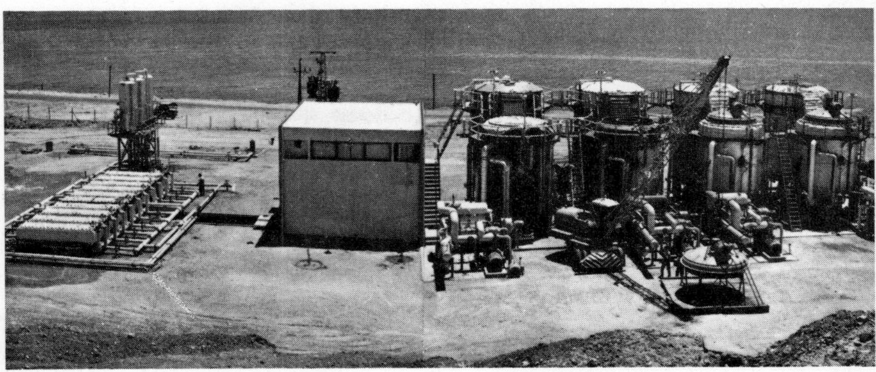

The Economics of Desalination

Clearly there is no point in trying to desalt the sea if the fresh water produced proves so costly that no one will be willing to buy it. Of course this is not so: if it were, the millions being spent on desalination research around the world today would never have been sanctioned. Research on this huge scale is based on the assumption that even if desalted water is expensive today, the results of this research will make the price competitive

Estimated comparative water costs for desalination plants of 22,500 m³/day capacity. Low- and high-cost utilities have been used as examples in compiling the chart and are reflected in the extremities of the horizontal ranges. The low costs are those of large nuclear reactor schemes that generate electricity and use low-pressure steam in distillation plants. The high costs are those of small and medium-sized plants of the type currently being installed. The water costs include allowances for direct raw materials, plant-operating materials, labor and supervision, maintenance, depreciation, interest on capital, and insurance. A working year of 292 days is assumed. Of the plant designs, only MSF has been proved a commercial proposition. The estimates for the secondary refrigerant process are based on a detailed design study and those for reverse osmosis are based on designs that require pilot plant studies. In general, costs will lie at the higher end of the range, because low-cost utilities are not available at this plant size. Steam costs are usually higher (except for "waste" steam) than electricity costs and so the lower end of the range for power-consuming processes must be compared with the higher range limits for distillation processes. The effectiveness of secondary refrigerant and reverse osmosis at low salt concentration feeds are clearly shown. Optimistic (1) and pessimistic (2) designs are shown.

Present MSF
Advanced MSF
Secondary refrigerant 10°C seawater
Secondary refrigerant 27°C seawater
Secondary refrigerant 10°C brackish water 0.5% salt
Reverse osmosis—seawater
Reverse osmosis—brackish water 0.5% salt
Electrodialysis—0.5% salt
Electrodialysis—0.25% salt

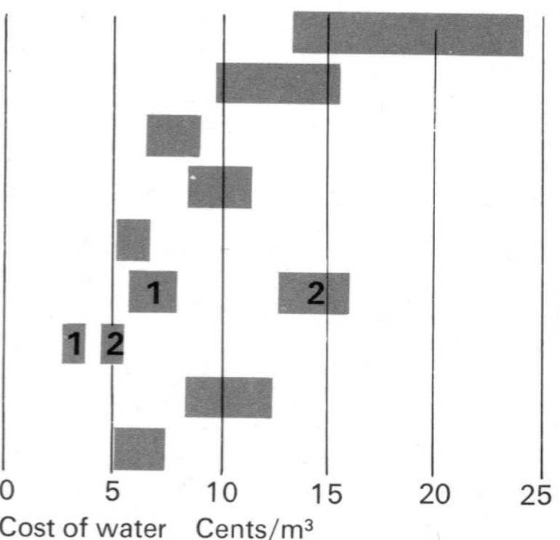

tomorrow. In fact a great deal has already been achieved in this direction.

First we should remind ourselves of the cost of water supplied today by conventional methods. Of course this varies greatly. In the United States the average cost has been quoted as being approximately $3\frac{1}{2}$ cents/m^3. In the United Kingdom it is in the region of 6 cents/m^3. Not only the cost of water, but its value too, varies, depending on the use to which it is put. It has been officially stated that in Israel a water cost of 11 cents/m^3 is economic to the farmer of cash crops. Yet in Chapter 1, we saw that in the water-short region of the southwestern states of America, irrigation agriculture adds only about 4 cents to the farmer's pocket for every cubic meter of water supplied. We also saw that in the same region every additional cubic meter of water made available to the industrialist enables him to earn at least $2.50. The cost of water produced by desalination processes varies even more widely and it is not easy even to make comparisons, because two of the major cost components—interest on capital, and the cost of energy used—themselves vary greatly. Interest may be as low as 4 per cent or as high as, perhaps, 10 per cent; the energy may be the "free" exhaust steam of a nuclear power plant, or electricity at 1 cent/kWh.

Desalinated water is still relatively expensive. The Freeport LTV plant produces water at 27 cents/m^3 and prices vary from this to 10 cents/m^3, which is the cheapest desalinated water actually produced at the present time. Research is directed toward reducing costs, and joint nuclear-power and desalination plants would seem to hold most promise for the future. At the moment engineering of natural freshwater resources remains the cheapest method of supply and it is only in certain arid regions of the world that desalination provides an economically viable solution to the water shortage problem.

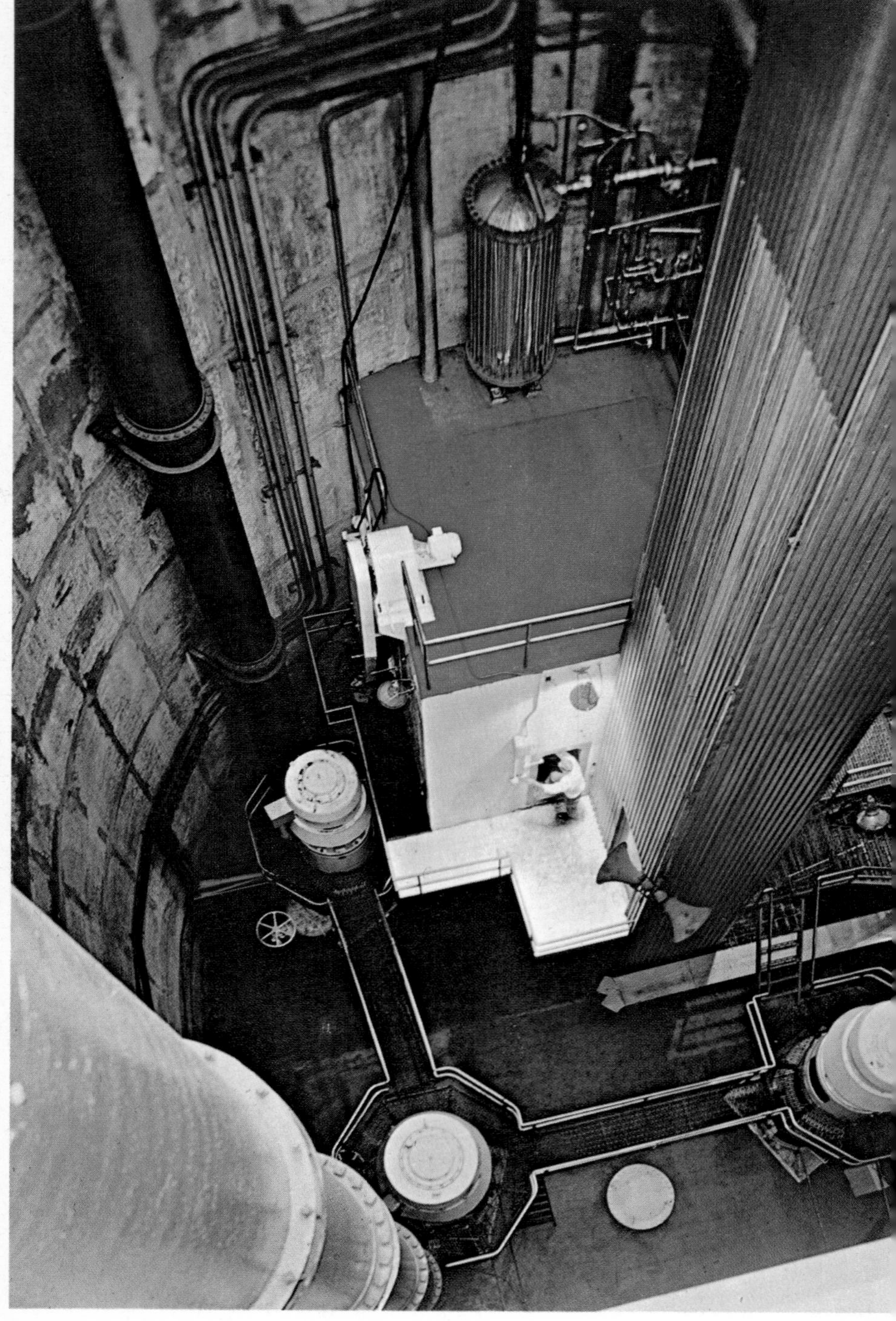

7 Purifying Water

Water is rarely pure. Though the water that circulates in the hydrologic cycle is distilled by natural evaporation, even as the rain falls it dissolves carbon dioxide from the atmosphere.

Natural Water

When a river flows through peaty moorland it picks up traces of organic acids and sometimes ammonia. Groundwater takes various substances into solution from the soils and porous rocks through which it percolates, even sulfuric acid from high sulfate clays, or the commonly found bicarbonate of calcium, formed when dissolved carbon dioxide (CO_2) reacts with chalk or limestone. Other substances found naturally in water include compounds of magnesium, sodium, potassium, iron, manganese, phosphorus, and silicon, and these are variously found as carbonates, sulfates, nitrates, chlorides, bromides, fluorides,

To prevent pollution of rivers that supply water-purification plants, used water (containing industrial waste and domestic sewage) undergoes sewage treatment before discharge. Some idea of the scale of this operation is shown here at the Nashville Central Sewage Treatment Plant, Tennessee, where used water arrives at an underground chamber and is conveyed by powerful pumps to the activated-sludge sewage plant (of 200,000 m^3 dry-weather capacity) at the surface.

and iodides. Fortunately the concentrations of all these substances in natural fresh water rarely make it unpalatable or otherwise unsuitable to drink, though a high CO_2 content can render water corrosive enough to dissolve lead, forming poisonous compounds. Dissolved carbonates and sulfates are responsible for the "hardness" of water; this constitutes no danger to health, but the consequent scaling of pipes and boilers may be troublesome where the hardness, in terms of calcium bicarbonate content, exceeds 0.02 per cent.

The fluorine content of drinking water can affect the dental health of man. People who regularly drink water containing less than 0.0001 per cent of the element fluoride show a greater incidence of tooth decay. The optimum concentration in water for healthy teeth is 0.0001 to 0.00015 per cent, whether the fluoride ion is naturally present or artificially added. Discovery of the beneficial dental effects of fluoride resulted from observation of changes in the appearance of teeth in persons who, from birth, had consumed water containing too much fluoride (0.00025 per cent or more). The manifestation of this too high level is known as *dental fluorosis* (see page 156), known earlier as mottling. Several other causes of similar discoloration of teeth exist, however, that are not related to the fluoride ion.

More than 0.0003 per cent of iron in water can cause brown stains in washbasins and baths, and on washed clothing; and over 0.0002 per cent of manganese results in the coating of the interior of pipework with an objectionable black slime. Natural water exists with high concentrations of sodium chloride along with other salts, both in the sea and in brackish groundwater. Desalination does not effect the removal of every trace of salt. This is not a serious drawback, because up to 0.02 per cent NaCl can rarely be tasted, and concentrations as high as 0.14 per cent can be tolerated—some public supplies of natural origin in Essex, England, contain this relatively high concentration of common salt.

The Problem of Pollution

The pollution of fresh water by human action was hardly known before two events of the most far-reaching significance took place in quick succession. One was the Industrial Revolution in Europe; the other was the invention of the modern waterborne sewage system and, in particular, of the water closet. Out of the first grew the problem of water fouling by industrial waste; from the second erupted the menace of bacteriological pollution.

Before waterborne sewage systems became general, it was the land that was fouled, and once fouled it usually remained fouled. The system of waterborne sewage had the theoretical advantage that waste matter was carried physically away and became innocuous, partly by dilution and partly, in the case of vegetable matter, by bacteriological action. The ancient Romans' sewage system worked on this principle and was entirely successful because the water flowed continuously through the city drains and was thousands of times in excess of the waste matter it had to carry. The effluent was therefore diluted to the extent of being harmless even before it ran into the river Tiber.

The rapid and uncontrolled growth of trade effluents that followed the Industrial Revolution in Europe soon resulted in chemical pollution overtaking dilution in stretches of river directly below large industrial centers. Agricultural pollution by fertilizers, insecticides, and pesticides also increased, and pollution by human sewage overtook bacteriological action in the growing urban areas of high population density. Many rivers in industrial areas thus became chemically poisoned, while in nonindustrial centers of population they became carriers of waterborne disease. Since rivers were the primary source of water for human consumption almost everywhere, pollution suddenly became a vital public problem. In England a Royal Commission on sewage disposal was set up in 1868, and eight years later the British Parliament passed the River Pollution Prevention Act, which became the model for similar legislation the world over.

Industrial pollution by directly toxic substances such as phenols, cyanides, and salts of chromium and lead, is now rare; legislation has seen to that. Pollution by the bacteria of disease, caused chiefly by waterborne domestic sewage, is controlled by water treatment. In addition there is pollution by two categories of nontoxic substances—those that can subsequently become harmful as a result of chemical or biological decomposition, and those that render the water aesthetically unpleasant or otherwise unacceptable for domestic use, or chemically and/or physically unsuitable for certain specific industries. Domestic considerations include color, taste, smell, turbidity, the presence of minerals causing digestive disorders, and the concentration of substances, such as fluorine and iodide, necessary for general health. Nontoxic industrial waste is exemplified by the effluents of coal-washing and china-clay plants, and by distillery waste. Sometimes, heat passed into water at power stations also has to be considered. In recent years two new forms of water pollution have arisen. One is fouling by detergents, the other is radioactive pollution. Neither is wholly removed by established water treatment processes, and both constitute a growing problem. Some public water supplies, after treatment, have been known to have a detergent content as high as 0.0001 per cent. And while nontoxic detergents do not appear to affect health, this is not a proven fact.

Perhaps the most worrying aspect of pollution control in the modern world is the rate of growth in the volume of waterborne sewage of which authorities have to dispose. American experts

Left: dental decay, common in persons drinking nonfluoridated water, i.e. less than 0.00005% fluoride. Center: healthy teeth, typical of persons drinking naturally or artificially fluoridated water, i.e. 0.0001 to 0.00015% fluoride. Right: dental fluorosis—healthy teeth, but poor in appearance (mottled)—caused by consumption of natural water containing too much fluoride (0.0006 to 0.0008%).

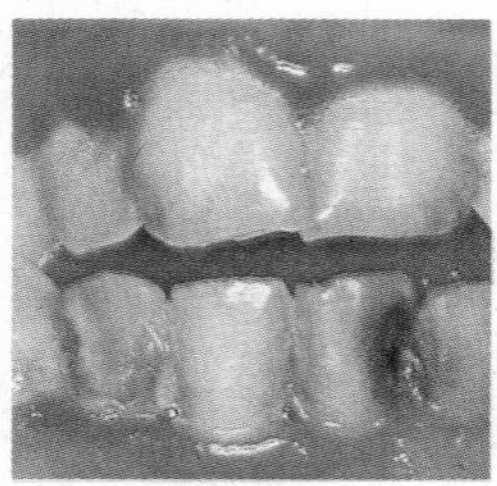

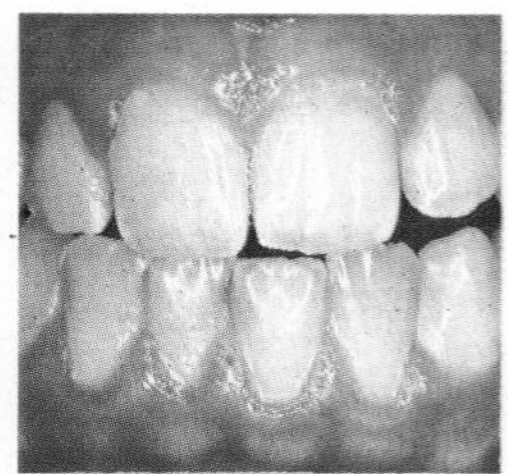

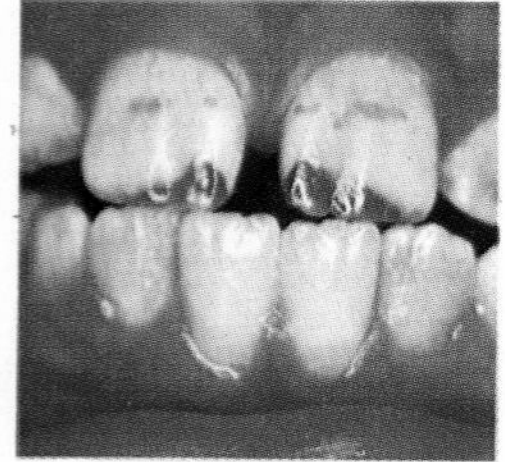

have said that the waste-bearing waters from domestic, industrial, and agricultural sources in the United States will reach a total of about 3000 Mm^3/day by the year 2000, representing an increase of about 400 per cent in 50 years. One recent problem has been the influx of nitrate into rivers and lakes. This chemical, produced by bacterial action in sewage effluent or washed directly from fields treated with nitrate fertilizer, encourages the rapid growth of algae (waterborne plants seen as green scum on ponds), which decay and cause more pollution. The problem is particularly serious in America, where Lake Erie—one of the Great Lakes—has been described as being "on the brink of a biological catastrophe" owing to an accumulation of rotting algae and organic wastes. Possible solutions to this problem, which has also affected several lakes in Switzerland, are massive effluent treatment schemes and restrictions in the use of nitrate fertilizer.

The Quality of Drinking Water

The maximum permitted concentrations of various substances in public water supply is controlled throughout the world by legislation and varies to some extent from country to country. The general concensus is summed up in the table shown on the next page.

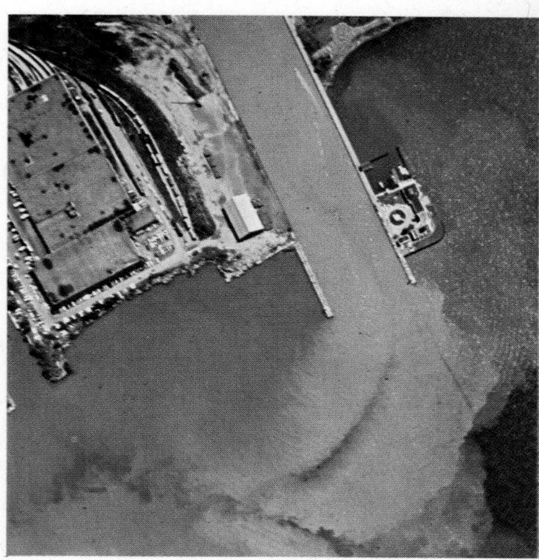

The increase in waterborne pollution during recent years has precipitated a biological crisis in some rivers and lakes. Effluent, discharged into Lake Erie, USA, threatens the balance of animal and plant life and renders the water unsuitable as a source for domestic water supply.

Substance	*Maximum percentage permissible in public water supplies*
Carbon dioxide	0.002
Carbonates of sodium and potassium	0.015
Chlorides	0.025
Chlorine (free)	0.0001
Copper	0.0003
Detergents	0.0001
Fluorine (as fluorides)	0.00015
Iron	0.00003
Lead	0.00001
Magnesium	0.0125
Nitrates	0.001
Phenols	0.0000001
Sulfates	0.025
Zinc	0.0015
Total solids in suspension	0.05

Natural water is often alkaline, sometimes slightly acidic. Alkalinity is usually due to dissolved calcium bicarbonate or other compounds of the base metals. Acidity is due either to dissolved carbon dioxide or to organic acids originating in peaty land. Sulfate acidity is sometimes acquired by rain falling through industrially polluted air. Some water treatment processes themselves render water slightly acidic. While there is no reason why water of low acidity should not be drunk, opinion favors a low alkali content and it is the aim of most public authorities to supply water with a pH value of either exactly 7 (neutral) or very slightly above. Comparatively small ranges of acidity or alkalinity of solutions are measured on the pH scale, numbering from 1 to 14; pH 7 represents a neutral solution and counting down from this point denotes increasing acidity; counting up represents increasing alkalinity.

While it is rare, today, due to the almost universal treatment of public supplies, for piped water to be contaminated, the list of diseases that water is capable of carrying is alarming. Among waterborne bacterial diseases are cholera, typhoid, paratyphoid, bacterial dysentery, and gastroenteritis. Virus diseases known to have been passed on by water include jaundice and, more rarely, polio. Biological diseases carried by water include amoebic dysentery and parasites such as tapeworms and flukes. The list is formidable; but more significant than the number or variety of these diseases is the fact that when they are found in water the root cause is almost invariably contamination by sewage.

The Testing of Water

The protection of water from pollution of all kinds begins and ends with physical, chemical, and biological examination. Many of the standard tests are simple and direct, such as checks for color, clarity, temperature, taste, and total solids content. More sophisticated physical tests include those for pH value

Dissolved oxygen in water can be quickly measured with a Mackereth electrode, shown in use below. The unit, which is submerged during operation, consists of a lead electrode sheathed in a polythene membrane. Oxygen gas diffuses through the membrane and reacts with the electrode to produce a current proportional to the gas diffusion rate. A microammeter, which measures the current, is calibrated to show the percentage saturation of dissolved oxygen.

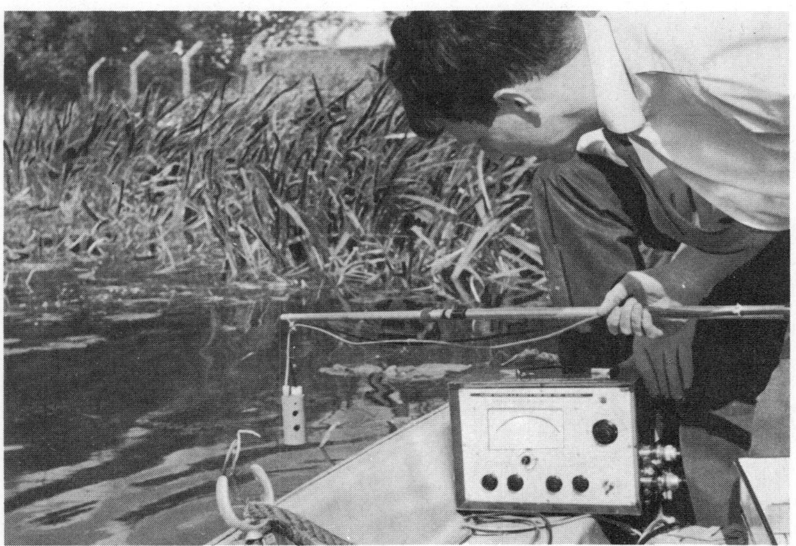

and for electrical conductivity. Chemical measurements normally carried out for public water supply include the water's content of nitrogen and oxygen (indicators of organic pollution), of calcium carbonate (giving the water's relative hardness), of chlorine (widely used in the sterilization of water), of fluorine, iron, manganese, lead, copper, and zinc. The presence of radioactive isotopes must be investigated and, if necessary, measured. Three important routine checks remain: of these the first is the measurement of the *biochemical oxygen demand*; the second is a bacteriological test of the content, if any, of human intestinal bacteria, known as the *coliform count*; and finally there is a biological check known as the *algal count*, which measures the microscopic plant and animal life, as distinct from bacteria and viruses, present in the water.

Under natural conditions the various living organisms in large amounts of water comprise a balanced community in ecological equilibrium. Clear fresh water is usually saturated with dissolved oxygen. Aquatic animal life consumes oxygen, and produces free carbon dioxide and waste matter. Waste matter is rapidly oxidized, partly by chemical action, partly by aerobic bacteria, in both cases the dissolved oxygen being further depleted. Simultaneously, aquatic plant life reoxygenates the water, consuming dissolved carbon dioxide and salts from decaying animal waste.

When water is polluted by unnatural causes, dissolved oxygen may be used up in the self-purification process faster than it is replaced. Eventually lack of oxygen encourages the action of anaerobic bacteria, which, instead of oxidizing, and thereby purifying, waste matter, start the process of putrefaction. When this process gains the upper hand the water turns foul. The presence of toxic substances also inhibits the action of oxidizing bacteria, so upsetting the natural balance. To establish the "oxygen balance" of water, the biochemist measures the biochemical oxygen demand, which is defined as the weight of oxygen absorbed by a given sample of water in five days at 20°C.

The existence of minute concentrations of pathogenic bacteria in water can render it dangerous to health. However it is virtually impossible to detect, let alone measure, such low concentrations by direct observation. Many of the bacteria and viruses involved cannot even be seen through the optical microscope. Human excreta contains thousand of millions of nonpathogenic bacteria per gram, the main species present being *Escherichia coli I*, a natural inhabitant of the healthy intestine, which can be seen under the microscope. Detection and measurement of the presence in water of the natural intestinal bacteria provides an immediate indication of the possible presence of pathogenic bacteria.

The coliform count is defined as the number of *E. coli I* bacteria present per 100 ml. of water. Only if the count is zero can the water be used for public supply. A count of 1 or more is taken as a positive indication of fecal pollution and the inherent risk of disease. Though the proportion of pathogenic to nonpathogenic bacteria is unlikely to exceed one to a million, which means that a coliform count of 1 indicates a possibility of one bacteria of disease-carrying bacterium in 100 m^3 of water, such water is considered polluted and should not be distributed in a public supply system without prior sterilization.

Water Treatment

We have seen the many ways in which water may be unsuitable for domestic use or for industry, either because of natural impurities or as a result of industrial or domestic pollution. As pollution of otherwise potable natural supplies is widespread today, though the control measures now imposed

The degree of pollution by pathogenic bacteria is based on a count of Escherichia coli (the most common intestinal bacteria) per unit volume of water. Shown is a nutrient plate that has been inoculated with a sample of the water under test. Colonies of E. coli have grown and those with a golden metallic sheen are counted; the total is called the coliform count.

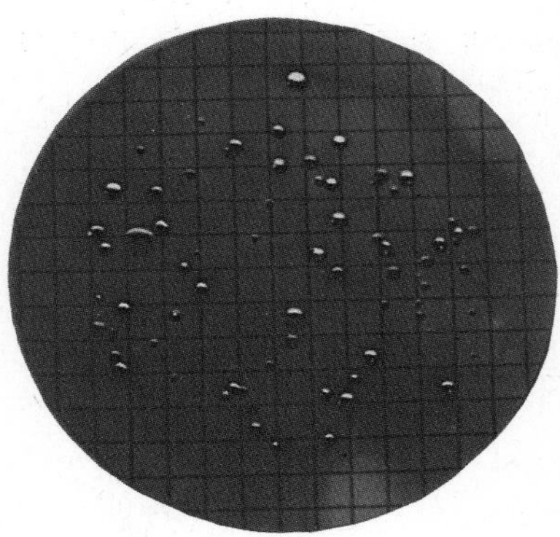

almost everywhere are beginning to reduce this, water supply undertakings must treat all water before distribution.

The term *treat* here is a very wide one, embracing a whole range of processes. The simplest method of all is treatment by large-scale open storage, reproducing the natural conditions that result in the self-purification of water. Water treatment techniques include screening and straining, sedimentation, coagulation and flocculation, filtration, aeration, and sterilization. To this list can be added further processes for the removal of color, taste, and odor, to make water aesthetically acceptable to the consuming public. In addition, water supplied to industry may have to be softened and demineralized. And for general advantage we should add measures for the elimination of corrosive action and for incrustation control.

The first step in the treatment of water is the removal of floating or suspended debris and living organisms, possibly including fish. The simplest screens, used where river, lake, or reservoir water is diverted to a waterworks intake, consist of vertical bars of about 2 cm. diameter, at between 6 and 10 cm. spacing. For finer screening, down to about 5 mm., rotating drums or continuous bands of perforated materials are used, water jets being directed to wash the screened material into a waste trough. Fast gaining favor is a development of the drum screen called a *microstrainer*, which utilizes a very fine mesh of stainless steel wire having as many as 25,500 apertures per cm^2. A microstrainer drum of 4 m. diameter and 4 m. long can pass about 1600 m^3 of water an hour and will strain out a great deal of extremely fine suspended matter, including virtually all plankton and algae.

Sedimentation

When water stands still, or nearly still, suspended solids sink to the bottom, forming a sediment. In water treatment plants, large shallow basins are used to arrest the flow of water sufficiently for natural sedimentation to take place before the water is drawn off. In theory one has only to calculate the rate of fall of the sediment—which depends on the density and size of the particles—and to make the basin large enough, and the flow therefore slow enough, for all suspended matter to fall out of suspension before the water has completed its passage. In practice there are many complications. Turbulence inhibits settlement of fine particles, and to avoid it may require a slower water velocity than the theoretical rate of settlement indicates. Another practical problem is the difficulty of ensuring an even flow through any large volume of water. When water enters a simple basin at one end and is drawn off at the other, the natural tendency is for a relatively narrow stream of water to take the shortest route between inlet and outlet, crossing the basin in a fraction of the theoretical time for an evenly spread flow. Baffles may help to solve this problem, though by deflecting the water up or down or sideways they may themselves cause turbulence and so partly defeat their own purpose.

Engineers have designed sedimentation basins of many kinds and it has been found that to be effective they almost invariably need to be about three times as large as indicated by calculation. Nor will a design that proves effective under one set of conditions necessarily repeat its performance in a different situation. Some of the particles found suspended in natural water are so small or of such low density that they will not settle even when the water is perfectly still. To aid sedimentation of such finely divided material, chemicals are used to induce them to form clusters. In most waters a spongy mass is formed, the induced action being known as *flocculation*. Most of the finer suspended particles found in water bear a negative electrical charge. When alum (aluminum sulfate) is added to alkaline water, aluminum

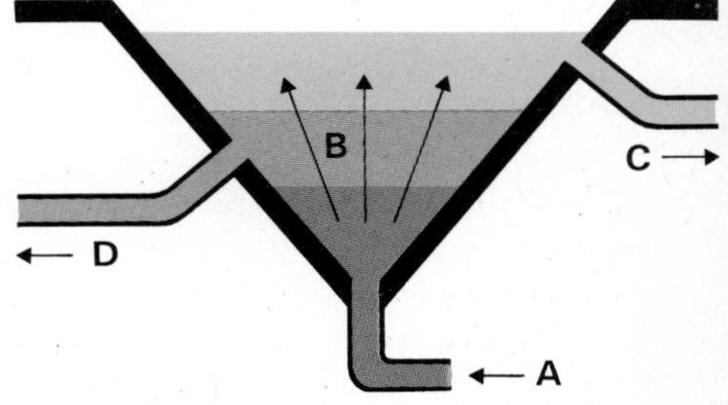

The principle of upward-flow sedimentation. Raw water, with added flocculants, flows from the apex (A) to the base of an inverted cone. As the cross-sectional area of the tank increases, the upward velocity of the water is reduced; where this balances the rate of fall of floc, a sludge blanket (B) is formed. This acts as a filter, and clear water is led off at (C). The sludge is pumped out at (D).

hydroxide is formed, together with sulfates of the bases present. Aluminum hydroxide, $Al(OH)_3$, in solution forms ions with a strong positive charge; these attract the negatively charged particles (and to some extent bacteria, some of which also bear negative charges), causing the suspended matter to coalesce. The *floc* formed can then be removed by sedimentation. Floc, however, is relatively light and sedimentation is consequently slow, requiring on average about three hours in a typical 3-m-deep basin.

Reduction in floc sedimentation time has been achieved in upward-flow tanks. It would appear anomalous for sedimentation, which involves the falling of particles by gravity, to take place in upward-flowing water. In fact the ingenious operation of upward-flow sedimentation tanks (which, in practice, are often of complex design) is simple enough in theory. In its basic form such a tank is an inverted cone; and, because the cross-sectional area increases rapidly from the apex (at the bottom) to the base of the cone (at the top), the upward velocity of the water is reduced as it rises. Somewhere in the tank there is a horizontal plane where the upward water velocity equals the average downward rate of fall of the floc. The result is the formation of a horizontal "blanket" of floc suspended in the water acting as a filter through which the upward-flowing water must pass. This process of filtration forces the negatively charged particles in the water into extremely intimate contact with the positive ions formed by the added coagulant. When the blanket becomes too dense it is removed by pumping out.

Alum is not the only flocculant used in water treatment. Sodium aluminate is also used, and in water, forms alkaline floc-forming substances. It is sometimes used in conjunction with alum for the coagulation of acidic water. Where iron is present in turbid water, alum may not remove it. In such cases it is usual to use ferric chloride, ferric sulfate, or ferrous sulfate, sometimes with other chemicals. The chemistry is complex, though basically similar to that of the alum process. The floc produced by alum can be made more dense, and so less liable to dispersion by turbulence, by the addition of "activated" silica—sodium silicate to which bicarbonate of soda, sulfuric acid, or chlorine has been added. Where sedimentation after coagulation by alum is unduly slow, as little as 0.00015 per cent of activated silica may speed the action significantly.

Sand Filtration

The bed of a sand filter in a water treatment plant is much more than a very fine strainer. Examination of such a sand bed in use reveals two distinct layers. The top one, only a few millimeters thick, is dominated by algae, plankton, and other microscopic plant life. These minute organisms decompose organic matter, consuming mainly nitrates, phosphates, and carbon dioxide, and releasing free oxygen. This gives the layer a powerful oxidizing, and therefore purifying, action. On the surface of this *autotrophic* layer is a skin consisting largely of inorganic particles, known by the German word *schmutzdecke* (which means a film, or "deck," of dirt—German scientists were the first to demonstrate how sand filtration actually works). The schmutzdecke acts as an extremely fine-meshed strainer.

Below the autotrophic layer, and extending as much as 30 cm., is the *heterotrophic zone*, where bacterial life predominates. Here nonpathogenic bacteria continue and complete the decomposition of organic matter in the water, reducing it to simple and unobjectionable inorganic substances. The sand bed thus acts as a highly efficient triple filter—physical, chemical, and bacteriological. So effective is it that at the time of a severe outbreak of river-borne cholera at Hamburg, Germany, in 1892, when some 8600 persons died, there was not a single case at Altona, a township situated a few kilometers downstream, although the town water was drawn from the river. The explanation was that Altona had recently installed slow sand filters through which the polluted water was passed. This type of filter was the first known reliable means of obtaining a sizable supply of pure water from a polluted supply.

In practice such a filter consists of a large shallow basin in which about one meter of sand rests on a gravel base, beneath which is a system of collector pipes and channels. Filtration takes place entirely by gravity percolation at a rate of about 0.15 m^3 per square meter of filter bed, this being achieved with a clean bed by maintaining the water level about 10 cm. above the sand surface. As the schmutzdecke grows steadily more dense the water level must be raised to maintain the rate of filtration. When the water depth is about one meter it is time to clean the sand bed. This is done by draining off the water and scraping off the top 2 cm. of sand; when the sand layer becomes unworkably thin, fresh sand is spread on top. Slow sand filter basins are relatively large, 100 m. × 40 m. being a typical size. Cleaning, which is nowadays carried out by a custom-built

A typical rapid gravity filter. Flocculated water enters at (A) and passes through a sand bed (B) and a layer of pebbles to the collector pipe system (C). The flow controller (D) maintains a steady discharge at different heads of water and varying degrees of sand fouling. The filter bed is cleaned by a compressed-air blast—via pipe (E)—which separates the sand particles, followed by a backwash of clean water (dotted line). Rapid gravity units operate at an average filtration rate of 4 m^3/m^2 of filter per hour, but this can be increased where pretreatment of water is more extensive.

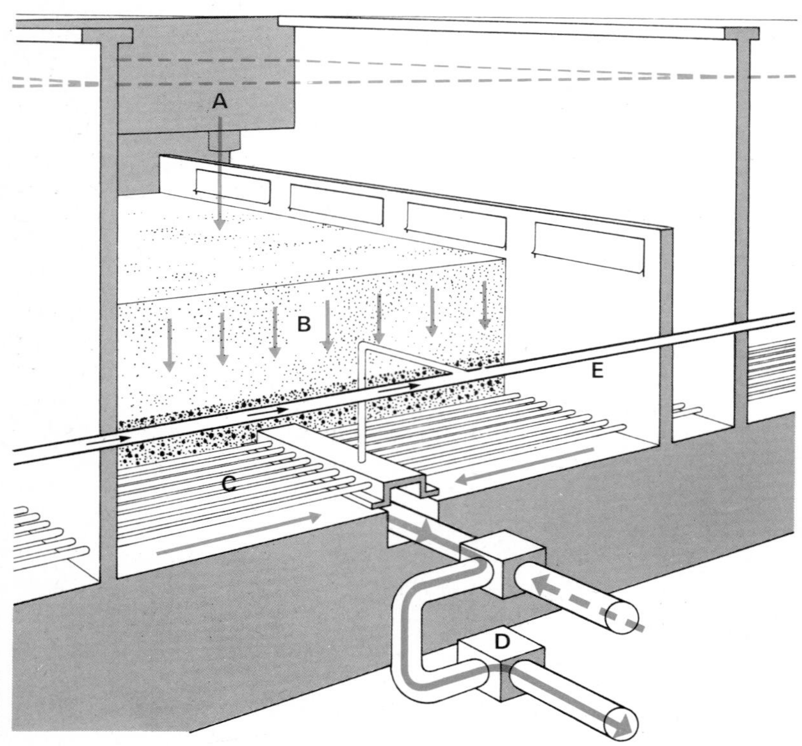

machine, is generally necessary every two to three months. A particular and useful characteristic of the slow sand filter is the establishment within it of a biochemical equilibrium that results in a water supply of uniform purity despite considerable variations in the quality of the incoming supply.

Slow sand filters are expensive to build and maintain, and due to the slow filtration rate they have to be inconveniently large. The rapid gravity sand filter was developed as an alternative, and it filters at a rate 20 times faster than the slow sand filter. Its mode of action, however, is not quite the same. No schmutzdecke forms at this high rate of flow, and no plant life can settle. Moreover the sand bed is cleaned by backwashing under applied air pressure, usually once in 24 hours. Although the rapid gravity filter has no autotrophic layer its action is partly physical, partly bacteriological. Unlike the slow sand filter, which filters pure raw water, the rapid type is designed for use with flocculated water.

While the rapid gravity filter is cheaper to install and operate than the slow sand type, and occupies far less ground space for the same output of water, it is considerably less efficient. Unlike the slow sand filter it cannot be guaranteed to provide a completely sterile effluent from heavily polluted water. A coliform count of 50 may be too high for it to remove entirely. The sand bed of a rapid gravity filter is usually between 0.5 and 1 m. thick. A typical tank size is 5 m. × 8 m. with a total depth of 4 m., this allowing for a maximum water depth of nearly 3 m. over the sand.

As a precursor to slow sand filtration, water may be passed through a pressure filter. This is essentially a rapid gravity filter enclosed in a steel pressure vessel, but containing sand of a much coarser grain. Water stays at mains pressure throughout its passage through the filter, and bacteriological action results in the removal of ammonia and any existing color.

Aeration

Water in contact with air dissolves the gases present until an equilibrium is set up. At normal temperature and pressure the final oxygen content is approximately 18 times that of carbon dioxide. Oxygen is a powerful purifying agent, and therefore forced aeration is beneficial to water having either a low oxygen or a high carbon dioxide content.

The simplest form of aerator is the cascade. Properly designed to break up the falling water and cause maximum turbulence, it can be extremely efficient. A single cascade with a 40-cm-diameter supply main will aerate 9000 m^3 of water a day, reducing the CO_2 content by 50–60 per cent and very substantially increasing the dissolved oxygen where the existing content is low. Weirs and waterfalls are natural cascade aerators, some weirs being especially designed for this role. When the water is made to cascade onto and then through a bed of coke, limestone, or anthracite, the CO_2 removal rate is further raised. Another form of aerator operates by spraying the water into the atmosphere through a large number of jets. Although this method is more efficient than the simple cascade, a high pressure head is required, making the process more expensive. A typical spray aeration plant with an output of 9000 m^3/day would require about 1000 jets.

Both types of aerator so far described require the pressure of the passing water to be broken, reducing to atmospheric pressure en route. Pumping is therefore necessary to bring the aerated water back to the original pressure. The injection aerator, which is sometimes designed to operate inside the top of a pressure filter, avoids this waste of energy. The water is simply sprayed under pressure into the enclosed space, fresh compressed air being circulated simultaneously.

Sterilization

Sometimes, where organic pollution is heavy, the source of raw water for a public supply is consistently suspect. To eliminate risk in such circumstances sterilization may be carried out after filtration, the killing agent being either chlorine or ozone. Ozone destroys bacteria by its powerful oxidizing action and has the added advantage of consistently reducing any color, taste, or odor in the water. It works rapidly, a dose of 0.0001 per cent destroying all bacteria, bacterial spores, and viruses within 10 minutes. The main disadvantage of the process is that ozone cannot be bottled and must therefore be manufactured at the waterworks. The process, which involves the passage of dried air through a powerful silent electric discharge, requires a supply of alternating current at not less than 4000 and preferably 20,000 volts, with a frequency of between 500 and 1000 cycles per second. This makes ozone treatment of water considerably more expensive than chlorination.

Chlorination is the commoner method of sterilizing public water supplies. Exactly how the chemical works is not known for sure. Though chlorine is an oxidizing agent, the low concentration that will sterilize most waters appears insufficient for oxidization to be the main killing process. Many scientists now believe that the hypochlorous acid formed when chlorine reacts with water inhibits the action of enzymes vital to bacterial

A water treatment plant designed to operate at an output of 9000 or 18,000 m^3/day. Raw water is screened at the river intake (A) and conveyed by way of pumps (B) to an upward-flow sedimentation tank (C). Chlorinated ferrous sulfate (flocculant) and lime slurry (softener and pH regulator) are added from supply tanks (D) and (E) respectively. Sludge from the sedimentation tank is pumped to a sludge lagoon (F) and the liquid recycled. Activated carbon (G) is added—to adsorb color-, odor-, and taste-producing impurities—as the water flows into the rapid gravity filters (H). One of the two chlorinators (I) supplies chlorine gas (sterilizer) to the contact tank (J) in proportion to water flow rate. Sulfonator (K) supplies sulfur dioxide for dechlorination. Powerful pumps (L) transfer water from the clear water tank to the mains supply (M).

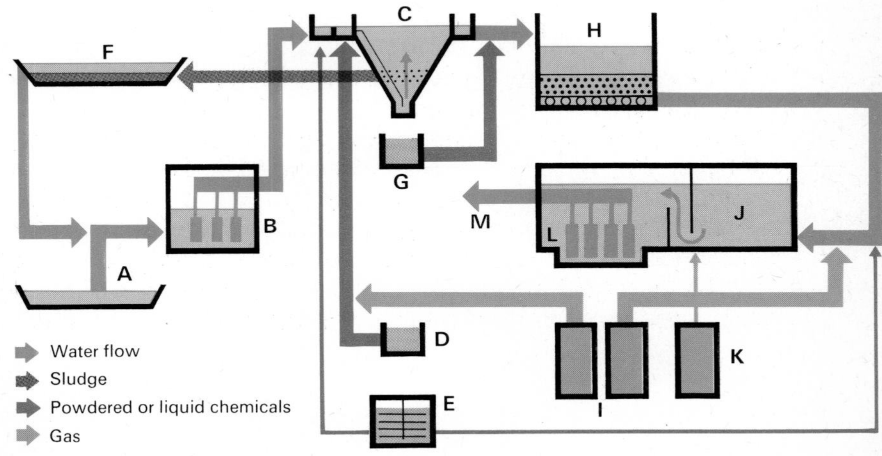

life. Chlorine is usually injected into water by precision apparatus that controls the pressure (and thus the flow) of the liquefied gas, meters it accurately, and mixes it with water under pressure. The mixture is finally injected into the raw water as it passes, at a controlled speed, through a closed conduit. The dosage of chlorine for effective sterilization depends to a great extent on the chemical content of the water. The presence of ammonia, either free or as compounds in organic matter, results in a chemical reaction that produces chloramines. While these have a mild sterilizing action, they are not to be compared in power with the hypochlorous acid produced when chlorine reacts with pure water. Consequently when ammonia is present in any form the chlorine dose must be increased so that free chlorine will remain after all the ammonia has been eliminated. The suspended matter in turbid water, organic and inorganic, also absorbs chlorine and may even prevent free chlorine penetrating to some individual bacteria. Water containing iron or manganese will neutralize some chlorine, forming insoluble chlorides. In all these cases, although greater than normal dosage might provide effective sterilization, it is more usual first to remove the offending substances by appropriate processes.

Chlorine does not sterilize water as rapidly or decisively as ozone. Some bacteria—that of tuberculosis, for example—are resistant to chlorine, as are certain bacterial spores and viruses. A dose that effectively reduces the coliform count to zero may not, therefore, destroy all pathogenic life in the water. Other factors that must be taken into account are the temperature and the pH value of the water. Either a drop in temperature or a rise in alkalinity results in a reduction in the killing power of chlorine in water.

The chlorine sterilization process most favored today is superchlorination followed by dechlorination. This ensures a thorough kill in a reasonably short contact period (30 minutes is normally considered adequate) and dechlorination, achieved by the addition of sulfur dioxide, provides flexibility. If so desired the chlorine can be entirely removed without the formation of any undesirable by-products. Alternatively, part of the original chlorine dose may be allowed to remain, providing insurance against subsequent light pollution within the distribution system. Where superchlorination is practiced, doses between 0.0002 and 0.0005 per cent are typical. It is virtually impossible to taste pure chlorine in water even up to a concentration of 0.0001 per cent, but chlorine reacts with other substances found in water and produces compounds that can be tasted and that may give rise to complaint. Superchlorination provides the answer here, too, as the high initial dose oxidizes and so destroys the offending substances.

The devices and processes we have discussed so far can be assembled in various combinations that will provide a public water supply acceptable to the most demanding health authority. But they may not always render the water aesthetically desirable in respect to taste, color, and odor. Where any or all of these are particularly troublesome, activated carbon is sometimes added as a fine powder or slurry. This adsorbs the odor-, taste-, and color-producing impurities and is itself removed during subsequent filtration.

Water Softening Processes

Hardness in water is due to the presence of calcium and magnesium bicarbonates (*temporary hardness*), which is deposited as scale when water boils, and the sulfates and chlorides of the same two metals (*permanent hardness*). Calcium carbonate, which is partly soluble in water, also contributes to permanent hardness to a limited extent. While hard waters are excellent for drinking, the dissolved salts inhibit lathering by soap—a drawback that has become less important since the introduction of synthetic detergents, because these lather in even the hardest water. The second important disadvantage of hard water is the deposition by it of scale on the inside of kettles, boilers, and pipes when the water is heated above 70°C. Scaling is a serious problem in many industrial processes.

There are two widely used methods for softening water in quantity. In the first, the addition of lime and soda results in the conversion of the soluble hardness compounds into insoluble substances that precipitate, and the formation of small quantities of innocuous soluble salts such as sodium sulfate or chloride.

The precipitate is removed by conventional means, usually coagulation by alum (aluminum sulfate) followed by passage through an upward-flow sedimentation tank, or by rapid gravity sand filtration.

The second and most modern technique for water softening is that of ion exchange. This process is based on the preferential "capture" of cations (e.g. Na^+, Ca^{++}, Mg^{++}) or anions (e.g. Cl^-, CO_3^{--}, SO_4^{--}) from solutions of salts by certain chemical substances. Natural greensand is one such substance but this has been superseded in use by synthetic ion exchange resins. The first types produced consisted of beads made up of cross-linked polystyrene chains containing active groups capable of attracting ions from solution. These polystyrene "gel" resins were pioneered in the late 1940s and are widely used today. Their disadvantage is a susceptibility to fouling by large organic molecules, which become lodged inside the hydrated bead. Newer macroreticular resins contain physical pores to facilitate absorption and desorption of organic molecules and colloidal ions. When water is required to be softened (as opposed to deionized—see later) it is passed through a base exchange unit. As the water flows through the polystyrene resin, calcium and magnesium (hardness-forming) ions are absorbed and an equivalent number of harmless sodium ions are released. The treated water thus contains as many ions as the ingoing water, but these are not of the scale-forming type. When the resin is completely depleted of sodium ions (and thus full of magnesium and calcium ions) the regeneration cycle is started. A strong salt solution is flushed through the medium, and the magnesium and calcium ions are replaced by sodium ions. The reconstituted resin is washed with distilled water and the unit is once again ready for use. The advantages of this process over the lime–soda process are that no sludge is produced and that regeneration and quality control can be made automatic.

Deionization (demineralization) is carried out where water is required to be of exceptionally pure quality. A cation and an anion resin are used in series. In the first unit the cations are replaced, not by sodium ions, but by hydrogen ions (H^+). The

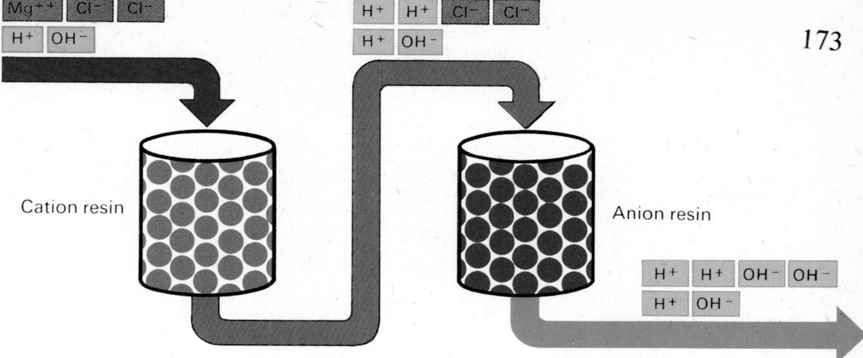

Above: demineralization of water using a two-bed ion resin system. The feed water is shown containing $MgCl_2$ (permanent hardness), of which the Mg^{++} ions are replaced by H^+ ions in the cation resin and the Cl^- ions are replaced by OH^- ions in the anion resin. The units are regenerated (i.e. restocked with H^+ and OH^- ions) by passage of acid and caustic soda respectively. Below left: a mixed bed unit in operation. This produces water of exceptional quality, because it travels between cation and anion beads many thousands of times during its passage through the unit. Below right: to regenerate a mixed bed unit, the lighter anion resin is first floated up by a water wash and the resins supplied separately with acid or caustic soda.

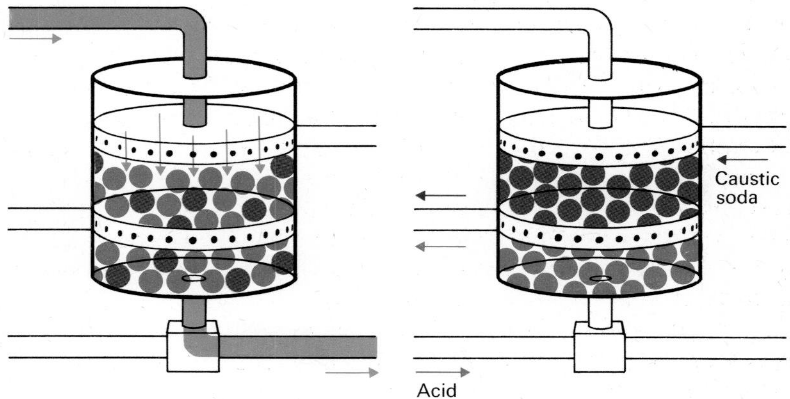

Below left: beads of a polystyrene gel resin (x 25); these are efficient but liable to deterioration in unfavorable conditions. Below right: beads of a macroreticular resin; these contain less exchange sites (taken up by physical pores), but are less susceptible to organic fouling and physical breakdown.

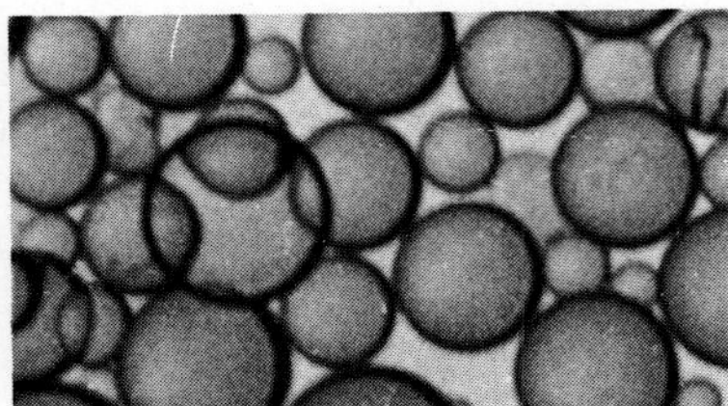

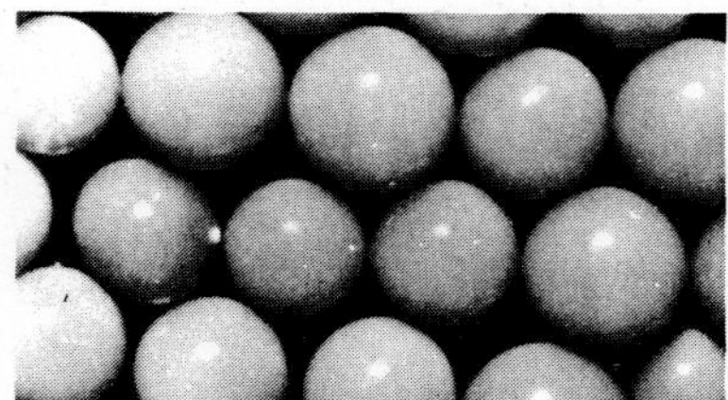

outflow (now acidic) from this section flows through the second resin unit, in which hydroxyl ions (OH^-) are substituted for anions. The resins are regenerated by sulfuric acid and caustic soda respectively. Mixed bed units, in which cation and anion resins are intimately mixed, are used to produce water of great purity (see page 173).

Detergents and Radioactivity

The only bulk water treatment process that removes synthetic detergents is slow sand filtration. Yet even this process, largely superseded today by cheaper rapid gravity or pressure filtration, retains at the most only 75 per cent of the detergent present, and considerably less where the concentration is initially low. The elimination of detergent from water is a growing world problem.

A partial solution may be afforded by control over the types of detergents permitted for general use. Some, known as "soft" detergents, are degraded by biochemical action and can therefore be removed by conventional water treatment processes. The West Germans lead the world here, having introduced legislation preventing the use of "hard" detergents. Although there is currently no such statutory control in other countries, biodegradable detergents are being introduced by enlightened manufacturers all over the world.

Another recent man-made pollution problem is that of radioactive waste. Atomic power stations, and similar installations that produce radioactive effluent, are bound by law to process this to within accepted safe limits of contamination before discharging it into rivers that supply domestic water treatment plants. Low- and medium-level radioactive effluent is first treated with flocculating chemicals and then passed to an upward-flow sedimentation tank. The sludge from this tank undergoes volume reduction by alternate freezing and thawing (ice crystals removed) and is then sealed in shielded disposal drums and dumped in the sea. The treated liquid effluent passes into an ion-exchange centrifuge—a circular wire basket layered with the sodium form of *vermiculite* (magnesium aluminosilicate), through which the liquid, entering at the center, passes under centrifugal force to collecting channels at the edge. The now virtually pure water passes to a storage and monitoring tank, and the lining of vermiculite is discarded and sealed in disposal drums.

Recycling Water

In the first chapter of this book we considered the uncomfortably rapid growth of water consumption in the modern world and the problems it poses for our hydrologists, engineers, chemists, and bacteriologists. We saw how a demand increase of, say, 10 per cent requires not only the finding of an additional 10 per cent of primary supply, but also a 10 per cent addition in water transportation, storage capacity, and treatment facilities. Treatment, as the reader will now appreciate, calls for extensive and varied plant and considerable space for the installation of that plant. Of course not every process described in this chapter will be necessary in any one application. But no one treatment is likely to suffice. And if the comparatively recent man-made problems of pollution by synthetic detergents and radioactivity are symptomatic of this age, who can say what new treatment problems the water chemist and bacteriologist may have to face in the future?

We should not, however, be too pessimistic. Every problem has an answer, and sewage treatment (which is similar in principle but more drastic than the water treatment processes we have described) is so well advanced that it has begun to play a significant part in alleviating the general water shortage. Some areas of the southeast of England today rely on river water over half of which originates as treated trade effluents and sewage. Industry, unable sometimes to obtain adequate high-quality supplies for its own use, paved the way by introducing demineralization processes, enabling it to reuse its own waste water. Man can do much the same with existing sewage purification techniques—it is only a question of plant capacity. So, in theory at least, by recycling the available resources, these can not only be doubled, but multiplied over and over again.

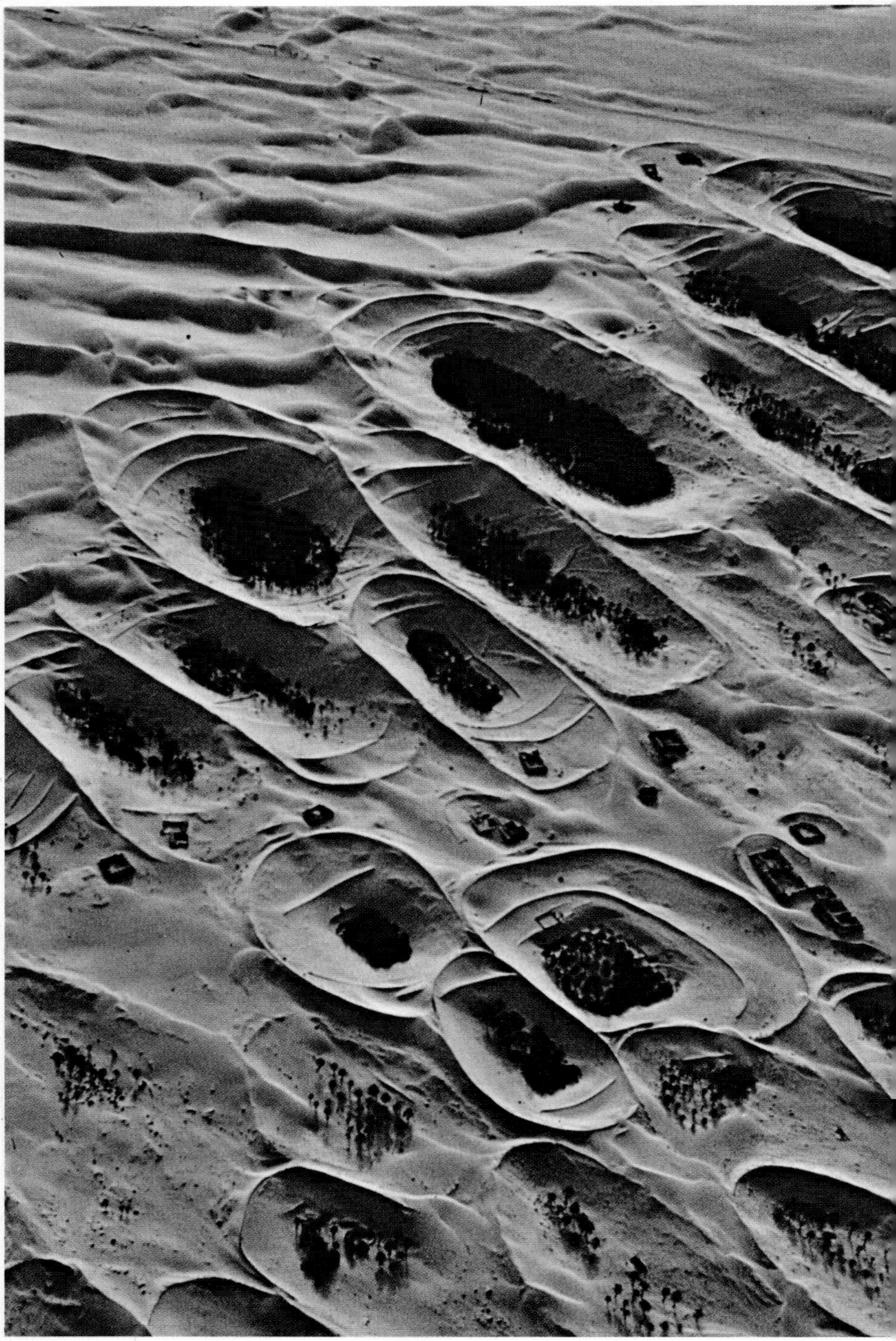

8 Future Water Resources

In this book we have seen how man has attempted to collect, purify, and make use of all the accessible sources of water in the world. There are, however, resources as yet untapped—the antarctic ice cap, for example; the many great rivers of the world that are still running to waste; the vast reservoir of the clouds. The sea is a potential source of fresh water, but large-scale desalination is still at the experimental stage. The projected schemes outlined in this final chapter show how the attempts to harness huge, but seemingly inaccessible, fresh-water supplies emphasize the water shortage problem and perhaps, in some cases, point the way to its ultimate solution.

The Making of Rain

Since earliest times the rainmaker has been treated, especially by the farmer, with deep distrust. When, in the 1940s, the "art" of rainmaking began to edge itself into the world of science, the new rainmaker at first fared no better. If he undertook to

Tapping unseen sources of water. Palm trees have been planted in deep, crater-like excavations in the sand dunes of Algeria, so that their roots may reach a subterranean stream.

produce rain and failed, he was run out of town. And if the rain fell, the farmer would probably maintain that it would have rained anyway. During the last 10 years, however, there has been conclusive evidence that the technique of cloud seeding, properly applied, can induce clouds to release their water earlier, and so in different areas, than would otherwise have been the case. So sure is the modern rainmaker of his art that, at least in Australia, he has begun to earn the confidence of those whose livelihood depends on timely rain. Just how widely the technique will be used in the future is not easy to predict, but it has become so certain a method of inducing clouds to shed their water that it can no longer be dismissed as being more chance than science. Nor need cloud seeding be confined to providing rain for crops at critical periods. It can be used today, in regions where the weather is of the right type, to increase the total annual rainfall of an area year after year. If the area is the catchment of a hydroelectric scheme, this can mean a regular increase both in the output of electricity generated and in the water available for domestic and industrial use.

How, then, does one set about seeding a cloud? The physics of the process has long been known. If either a very cold substance, or one with a crystal structure similar to that of ice, is introduced into a cloud of supercooled water droplets, ice crystals begin to form, and grow until they are too heavy to remain suspended in the atmosphere. Early experiments in Australia (1947) used Dry Ice (solid carbon dioxide) with considerable success, but such large quantities are needed that this could never have been practical for seeding large areas of cloud. Subsequent work has concentrated on the use of silver iodide smoke, for the silver iodide (AgI) crystal has a suitable structure and is found to act as an excellent "seed" for the formation of ice. In some parts of the world, where there are mountains 4000 to 6000 m. high, silver iodide smoke can be generated on the ground and carried up to the clouds by convection. But the introduction of the smoke into the clouds by aircraft is more reliable and, in flat country, essential. The smoke is produced by burning a solution of silver iodide in acetone in an apparatus suspended under the aircraft's wing. Light twin-engined planes are used and are capable of releasing about 1 kg. of AgI per hour. Clouds to be seeded must be chosen carefully, the crucial factor being their temperature. In practice it has been found that the top of the cloud must never be warmer than −10°C. Provided this is ensured, the yield of water will often exceed 250,000 m^3 per gram of silver iodide. The yield is two or three times greater than the rain that would precipitate naturally at the same time from the same clouds. As for long-term results, a series of carefully controlled experiments extending over several years in southwestern Australia has shown that in this area, where cloud formation of the required type occurs regularly, the established annual rainfall can be increased by between 25 and 30 per cent. Of more importance is that the additional rain can usually be induced when the farmer most needs it.

The economics of cloud seeding are as encouraging as the success of the technique itself. In average terrain the overall cost of an aircraft, including all operational expenses, aircrew salaries, seeding materials, and overheads, is about $75,000 a year, though this figure could be doubled in areas where unusual navigation or weather hazards exist. A single aircraft and crew

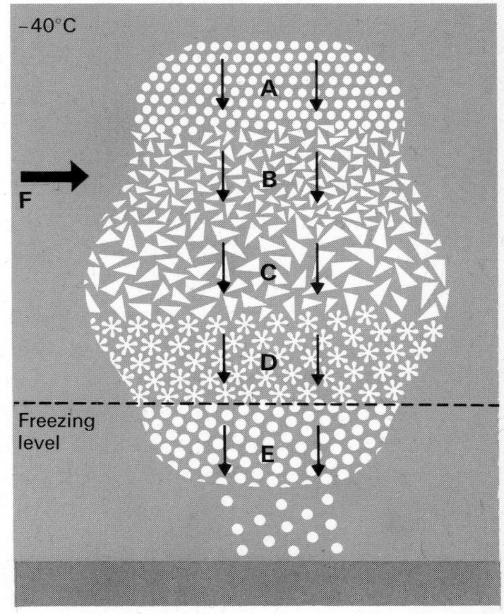

Rainmaking techniques are effective only on existing cloud formations and only on those clouds that extend above the −10°C level. The processes occurring naturally in such clouds have been proposed by the Swedish meteorologist T. Bergeron, and are shown opposite. The top of the cloud is thought to consist of supercooled water droplets (A) in equilibrium with small ice crystals (B). By coagulation large crystals (C) are produced, which coalesce to form snowflakes (D). Rain (E) is formed as these snowflakes fall below the freezing level. AgI crystals introduced at (F) are thought to provide sites for the formation of small ice crystals from supercooled water droplets and also facilitate coagulation processes lower down in the cloud.

can effectively seed an area of 25,000 km^2 throughout the year. The basic cost, in average country, would be as low as \$3 per square kilometer per year. Assuming the operation to be carried out in an area with the low annual rainfall of 20 cm., an increase of 25 per cent represents an addition of 5 cm. of rainfall a year, or 50,000 m^3/km^2. At a cost of \$3/km^2 this means pure fresh water at the fantastically low cost of 0.006 cents/m^3. In the case of cloud seeding for agriculture this is the only cost. In an estimate made for a 6000-km^2 tract of wheat country in the Mallee-Wimmera region of the Australian state of Victoria, where the crop yield is highly sensitive to the quantity and timing of rain falling between August and October, one aircraft inducing rain when most required can increase the value of the crop by about \$3 million. At a total investment of \$20,000 this is profit indeed. The same technique used to boost the annual rainfall of a hydroelectric catchment area would yield remarkably high profits for the water authority concerned. In a still incomplete long-term experiment over a hydroelectric catchment area in Tasmania, early figures have indicated that the cost of seeding the entire area can be paid for by a one-per-cent increase in mean rainfall. Any increase in precipitation above this one per cent represents profit without further cost. Judging by current experimental results, rainmaking is an example of that rare proposition, a gilt-edged investment with a high return.

Watering the Deserts

I have considered Egypt many times in previous chapters and have pointed out that this country would be barren wasteland, were it not for the river Nile. Yet the river Nile is not Egypt's only source of water. A glance at the map reveals a chain of scattered oases that would appear to tell a tale. In fact it is the tale of an underground freshwater "valley" running north–south, some 400 km. west of the river—a valley covering over 90,000 km^2. Like the other recently discovered aquifers in more western parts of North Africa, it is brimming with fresh water. Egypt has recognized its value and made it the basis of a little-publicized scheme to irrigate 400 km^2 by artesian well, with a planned expansion later to 1200 km^2. Not very many years ago no one dreamed that the water source of the oasis chain was so vast, and could yield so much water.

The deserts of Israel and Jordan could be supplied with fresh water by very large-scale desalination of the Mediterranean Sea. This idea, originally suggested by Mr. Edmund de Rothschild, writing in a mid-1967 edition of *The Times* of London, has been reviewed by Michael Ionides, an authority on the water resources of the Jordan Valley, and found to be a practical possibility. The river Jordan, which—with its tributary, the Yarmuk—supplies both countries, has an average daily flow of 2.5 Mm^3. Three desalination plants, with a combined daily output of 1.5 Mm^3 of fresh water, have been envisaged to supplement this supply.

Technically there is no problem. Desalination plants of 500,000 m^3 daily output are large by any standard, but American, British, and Soviet industry are all perfectly capable of designing and constructing them. The cost of water produced by such plant would lie somewhere between 6 and 8 cents/m^3. This sounds expensive but Israeli economists have stated that 8 cents/m^3 is not too high for cash-crop agriculture in Israel. The estimated cost today is not necessarily the final word. Commercial exploitation of the minerals removed from the desalted water is a possibility that might be feasible in a project as large as this, and might significantly reduce the cost of water produced. The actual cost should not be the only measure of desalted water's value in a world where industrially advanced countries divert huge sums to feed refugees or the victims of famine. It is cheaper sometimes to subsidize the desalination of water so that the needy can grow food for themselves.

The plant would necessarily be located near the sea coast, and this would create a problem. For Israel it would be adjacent to the rich farmlands in the south, but to share the water with upland Jordan would require expensive long-distance pumping. To avoid this expense, revised allocation of the water has been suggested. Instead of the two countries sharing the river Jordan's water on the one hand, and the desalted seawater on the other, it would clearly be more practical to give Jordan her share from the river, and supply all the desalinated water to the nearby Israeli farms. Would Israel agree to forego part of her natural source for the benefit of both; or would a vulnerable pipeline remain unmolested between these two countries? The main obstacle to the application of such a scheme would appear to be that of political mistrust.

Northwest Australia is a semidesert. The land is potentially fertile but lacks the water needed to grow crops. Along a 1600-km. stretch of the coast the average tidal range exceeds the 10 m. considered the minimum for economic exploitation as a source of power; and the coastal geography of the region is also well suited to the construction of tidal-power plants. Electrical authorities are not interested, because the area has virtually no population, and therefore no electrical demand. Port Darwin, the nearest small city, lies some 800 km. by land from the northern end of the strip of coast most favorable for tidal-power production. Perth is 1500 km. to the southwest of its other extremity. The tidal energy that could conveniently be converted into electrical power along this ribbon of coast is in the region of a million million units (1 TkWh.) a year, five times the total consumption of the United Kingdom. This power could be used to irrigate the dry but fertile land by desalinating seawater and pumping fresh water ashore. Calculation shows that the power could, in fact, provide an area of 75,000 km^2 with 50 cm. of irrigation water each year. In terms of food production this project has a vast potential, and in terms of return on capital cost it is economically sound. But the investment would necessarily be gigantic and the Australian government has other, less demanding schemes on which to spend. Perhaps the recent discovery of extensive iron-ore deposits in the area will shortly create sufficient immediate electrical demand to encourage ambitious speculators.

Coastal regions could also be supplied with fresh water from the air. J. L. Worzel and R. D. Gerard of Columbia University, New York City, have suggested that an on-shore condenser, supplied with cold seawater, would cool moisture-laden coastal winds sufficiently for condensation of fresh water to occur. A calculated output of 4000 m^3/day has been quoted for a plant on St. Croix, one of the Virgin Islands in the Caribbean Sea.

The Rerouting of Rivers

The diversion barrage, a means of rerouting a river to man's advantage, is demonstrated on the grand scale by a remarkable Soviet project. Two of Russia's major rivers, the Ob and the Yenisei, flow from the dry Kazakhstan uplands and Altai Mountains through the swamplands of the North, where rain is abundant, to the Arctic Ocean. Soviet engineers, studying this situation, have devised a brilliant and bold scheme that would enable $12\frac{1}{2}$ per cent of the water now flowing north to be diverted southward and used to irrigate great areas of the

The proposed scheme to irrigate over 10,000 km² of potentially fertile land of the central Soviet steppes involves damming the Ob and Yenisei rivers and diverting water to the south. A lake almost the size of Italy would be formed from the waters of the Ob and its tributary the Irtysh, and this, with additional supply from the Yenisei lake, would flow via canals to the Aral and Caspian seas.

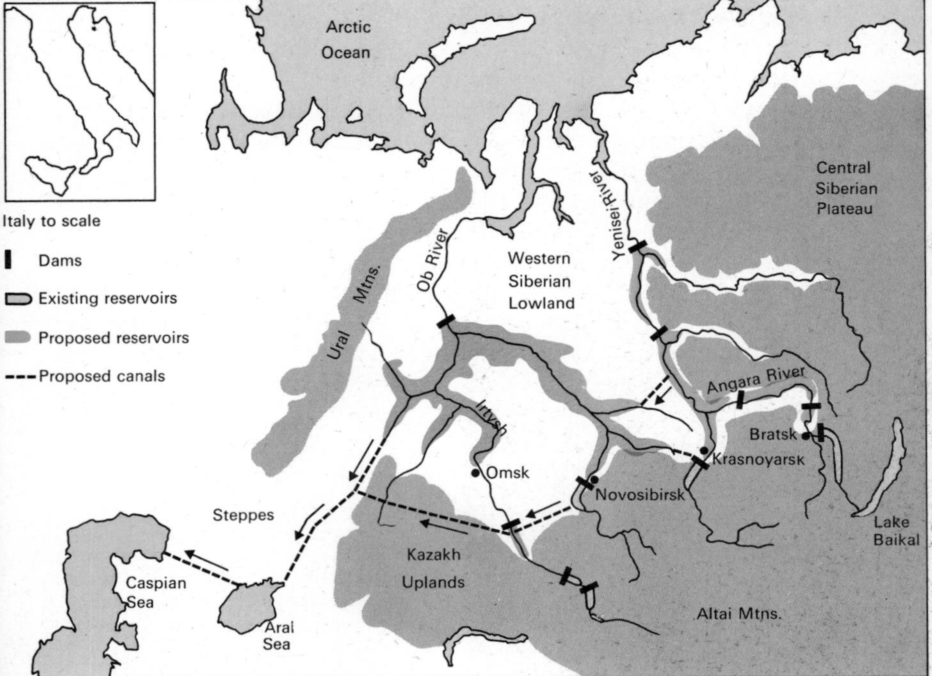

central steppes. The proposal includes the construction of a great dam across the Ob, just north of the point where its main tributary, the Irtysh, joins it, and the consequent formation of a multibranched inland freshwater sea almost the size of Italy. Another large man-made lake created by a huge dam across the Yenisei would then be linked with the eastern arm of the new Ob sea by canal. Canals would also connect the Ob sea, via the Aral Sea, with the Caspian Sea. Further long canals, running east–west, would link the Ob–Aral Sea canal with a new reservoir on the Irtysh and, further east, with an existing man-made lake higher up on the Ob. The Ob and Yenisei waters diverted south by this scheme would be sufficient to irrigate over 10,000 km^2 of potentially fertile land in Kazakhstan and Western Siberia. In terms of food production the scheme has a vast potential. It would also provide an installed electric generating capacity of some 70,000 MW.

Freshwater Stores in the Sea

One of the strangest hydrologic discoveries ever made was a pocket of pure fresh water in the sea off the Florida coast near St. Augustine, 100 km. north of Daytona Beach. This pocket, first reported in 1925, is about 30 m. in diameter and is located over a 40-m-deep depression in the ocean bed in an area where the average depth is 15 to 20 m. The fresh water issues from a

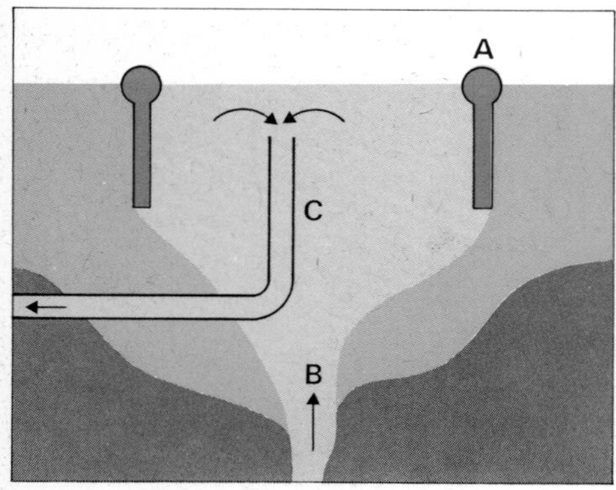

Left: the formation of a freshwater reservoir in the sea by placing a floating curtain (A) around a submarine spring (B). Fresh water (containing some salt) would be led away via a pipeline (C) to a shore pumping station. A similar system could be used to collect water from an Antarctic iceberg (shown right) at a projected water cost of 0.1 cent/m^3.

submarine spring at a rate estimated at 40 m^3 a second, or 3.4 Mm^3 a day.

This particular source of fresh water is a geological freak, but it may not be unique. It is unlikely that it will ever be used, but in theory its exploitation should not be technically difficult. All that is required is for a floating "curtain" to be moored over the submarine spring, forming a reservoir of fresh water that could be led, via a 4-km. trunk main laid just under the seabed, to a shore pumping station.

Perhaps the most tempting of all possible freshwater sources are icebergs—mountains of freshwater ice floating in the polar seas. A plan to use icebergs as a freshwater supply for American cities, the brainchild of John Isaacs of the American Scripps Institute, is theoretically straightforward and on paper seems economically worthwhile.

A selected iceberg is towed, via the favorable Humboldt current, up the west coast of South America until it slows down off Peru, then steered northwest in the path of other known currents that sweep in a great arc, via Hawaii, almost to the Californian coast. Arriving at Los Angeles the iceberg would be grounded offshore and surrounded by a 6-m-deep flexible floating "curtain" that would impound the fresh water as it melted. Now all that remained would be to pump the floating fresh water to the mainland, remove any salt that might have

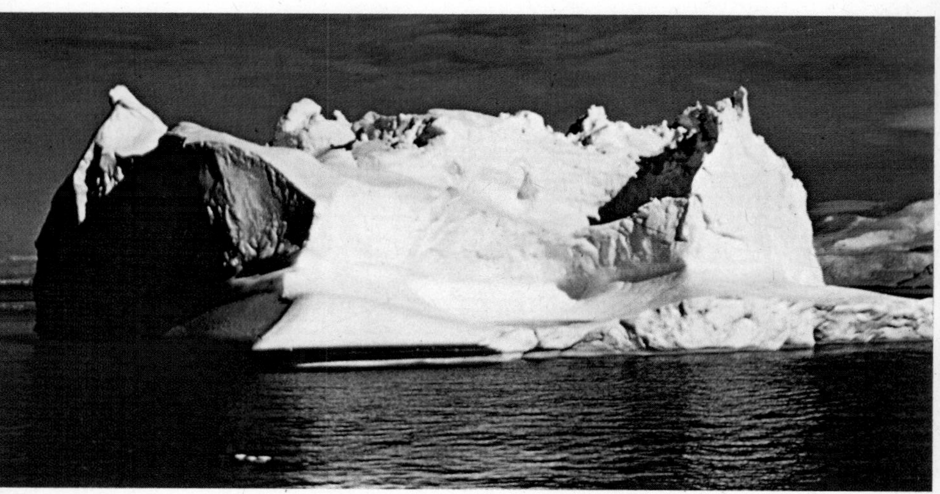

permeated it (a simple process, because the concentration would, at most, be very low), and finally pipe it into the local distribution system. The cost of such water would depend almost entirely on the size of the iceberg. In the Antarctic, where they are usually larger than in northern waters, an iceberg of the required size—i.e. 15 km. long, 1 km. wide, and 200 m. deep—would not be hard to find. One of this size could be brought to California by three oceangoing tugs. It would take a month to achieve a speed of two knots and the journey would take about a year, during which perhaps half the iceberg would melt away. Even half an iceberg of this size would yield about 1500 Mm^3 of fresh water, enough to supply Los Angeles for several months. Allowing $1 million for the hire of three tugs and their crews, and a further $½ million to cover handling the water at Los Angeles, the cost of fresh water delivered would work out at a modest 0.1 cent/m^3. Los Angeles is not buying this scheme; instead it will have the $500 million nuclear-power and desalination plant illustrated in Chapter 6. In the light of increasing world demand for fresh water, Mr. Isaacs' iceberg scheme may one day prove important, but not, it seems, in the immediate future.

Conclusion

Of the projects described in this chapter only a few are actually in operation. This is regrettable; but what is more important is that all of them are capable of success. The water crisis can be averted. The International Hydrologic Decade represents the greatest single step in this direction. The financial and industrial resources of many countries are contributing to this massive research program, whose aim is to guarantee world water supply for the present and foreseeable future. Technologically, therefore, man is equipped to meet the water shortage, but what is not clear is whether world governments and authorities are bold enough to grasp the fuller implications of the problem. If man does fail to take the steps today that will supply him with ample fresh water tomorrow, the failure, in the final analysis, will be a failure of management, and of management alone.

Postscript—Water Resources Planning in the 1970s

Riyadh, the desert capital of Saudi Arabia, possesses no source of surface water and the city had for some time drawn on upper ground water for domestic supplies and for irrigating local gardens. During the late 1960s the upper aquifers became polluted with sewage and to a great extent exhausted. Exploitation of the deep Minjur aquifer under the city was resorted to and water of a relatively poor quality was then pumped from a depth of 1200 meters.

In 1974 thé Saudi Arabian Ministry of Agriculture and Water commissioned a firm of consulting engineers to identify additional sources of fresh water for the city, whose population had been growing rapidly, throwing an increasing strain on services and in particular on the water supply system. For some years consumers had had to purchase water brought in by tanker at considerable expense during the hot summer months from May to October.

After nearly two years of intensive survey, drilling and test pumping backed up by desk studies the engineers, who had been asked to propose methods of increasing the city's water by 100,000 m^3 a day, reported three alternatives. The first was to draw additional water from the Minjur aquifer and to desalinate it before distribution. The second was to exploit the Wasia aquifer situated about 100 km. east of Riyadh, pumping the water to the city following normal water treatment. The third was to subject the Wasia water to full desalination before pumping it to the city.

The consultants found cause for concern in the further development of the Minjur aquifer. They estimated that the peizometric level would be drawn down some 100 m. in the first five years, affecting all existing wells at a cost which was not accurately predictable. There would also be a serious new problem of disposal of saline water from the desalination process. While the plentiful Wasia water would be cheaper without desalination, its quality was inconsistent and the consultants recommended this scheme with desalination, producing water at an estimated cost, at 1975 prices, of SR 3.30 per cubic meter. The engineers also recommended setting up of a pilot scheme to evaluate the relative merits, using typical Wasia water, of reverse osmosis and electrodialysis.

Early in 1976 the Saudi Arabian authority accepted the consultants' proposals with a single rider. Instead of extracting, desalinating and pumping 100,000 m^3 of water to Riyadh city, the engineers were asked to go ahead with a scheme to supply the capital with 200,000 m^3 of additional fresh water! This change made the scheme the largest single city water supply project ever undertaken, with the largest plant ever planned for the desalination of water for human consumption. The water to be extracted is, incidentally, fossil water believed to have been trapped underground for over 35,000 years. The estimated cost is $600 million at 1976 prices, and the project will take 5 years to complete.

The case of Riyadh is exceptional, but it underlines the case presented in the opening chapter of this book—that the world's water resources are immense and that the problem of water supply in relation to human growth is a problem of management, not of overall sufficiency. It is a problem of engineering and therefore a problem of cost. The countries of the middle east can have water in the desert because their oil has made them rich enough. Because they know their oil will not last for ever they are wisely spending huge sums on securing water while they have the cash to buy the costly engineering.

In Iran the government is using its oil revenues, backed by the

World Bank, to pay for engineering works designed, literally, to water the desert so that the abundant sunshine can be used to produce food. The country is fortunate in possessing a great river system based on the Tigris and its tributaries.

The Lower Khalis Project covers a huge area lying between 10 and 60 km. north of Baghdad. It involves construction of a new concrete lined irrigation system to replace and extend an old inadequate canal layout, including about 55 km. extension to the existing Khalis main supply canal to command about 50,000 ha. by gravity flow from the Diyala river. It also includes two pump stations on the Tigris river to supply about 7,000 ha., about 540 km. of branch and distributory canals, and approximately 1200 km. of other watercourses, all with related structures such as culverts, aqueducts and bridges. Also under construction is a land drainage disposal system, the extension and raising of a flood protection embankment along the right bank of the Diyala river, the installation of field drains and levelling of farmland throughout about 57,000 ha. within the Project area, the construction of about 300 km. of new all-weather feeder roads to connect villages in the Project Area to the main roads, the construction of offices, staff housing and related buildings for the Project Administration, and the provision of maintenance equipment, workshop machinery, vehicles and spare parts for the operation and maintenance of the Project.

Nor is this pursuit of new means for transferring water from its abundant sources to areas where it can profitably be made use of confined to the water-starved oil-rich middle east. Indonesia has the ingredients of the formula—a rapidly growing population, fertile land with insufficient water, water running to waste or otherwise unused, and oil to provide cash. So in central Java we find specialist engineers extending an old and inadequate canal system to irrigate 6000 ha. west of Jogjakarta, building a huge new pump station to feed water from the Kali Progo river into the new canals and backing the Project with the means of maintenance—roads, workshops and plant. And, in East Java, the Kediri-Nganjuk Groundwater Project covers the whole of the middle Brantas river basin in part of which a planned 730 tubewells should be capable of irrigating an estimated total of 56,650 ha.

In Nigeria the Ministry of Water Resources has embarked on an ambitious programme designed to use the country's valuable oil revenues to ensure that Nigeria's immense water resources are fully utilized so that she will never again suffer the crippling effects of drought experienced in the early 1970s. The Chad Basin Development Authority is at present engaged in the construction of a huge pumping station and 30 km. feeder channel to carry water for an irrigation scheme embracing 192,500 ha. —the first stage of the South Chad Project which, incidentally, includes the building and equipping of a 25 MW power station.

In parts of the third world not blessed with oil to meet the bill we find international organizations paying to provide water for hungry people.

In Ethiopia a two-year rural development study completed early in 1976 by a team of experts in a variety of disciplines has proposed an eighteen-year programme with immediate action on soil stabilization, the provision of domestic water supply and the strengthening of a regional water supply administration, followed by irrigation development and the construction of storage dams. The Study Report has been accepted by the Government and engineers have been appointed to set up six pilot projects for water supply in medium sized rural settlements in the Tigrai area and to establish a National Water Resources administration at Makalle. The new organization will undertake surveys of water resources, both subsoil and surface, for development. Meanwhile the International Development Association has earmarked funds for the construction of between forty and fifty similar water supply schemes throughout Ethiopia, based on the findings of the pilot projects.

By the end of 1975 the first successful harvest came off virgin land in the Afgoi-Mordile irrigation project west of Somalia's capital, Mogadishu. This project—the first controlled irrigation scheme implemented by the Somalis—draws hitherto unused water from the Shebelle river, and followed a feasibility study paid for by the United Nations. While the first harvest consisted of maize, rice, sorghum and groundnuts, it is planned also to produce cotton in future. The construction works, financed by the Government of Libya and the African Development Bank, included the building of a project village with its own electricity supply and tubewells to supply domestic water.

Other irrigation work currently in hand in Somalia includes a 200 Mm^3 offstream reservoir due for completion in late 1977, and studies for land drainage works for an existing sugar estate and for irrigation, drainage and infrastructural works for a proposed new sugar estate. It is notable that in Somalia, which has no oil, water management is directed towards the production of cash crops for export as well as for growing more food.

About 160 km. south east of Khartoum the Sudanese Rahad Irrigation Project has a similar objective. Designed to change some 1 million ha. of semi-arid desert into productive farm land from which cotton and groundnuts are to be the principal crops, the foreign exchange required for construction works is being provided by the World Bank, the Kuwait Fund and other international agencies. Works required to bring irrigation water from the Blue Nile river to the development area, some 83 km. away, were begun in 1975. They include a supply canal to convey water at the rate of 105 m^3/sec from a new pumping station on the river, crossing the river Dinder by siphon and discharging into the Rahad river where a new barrage and irrigation headworks are also being built.

Also under way in Sudan is a project to provide a drinking water supply for every village. There are huge areas in the Sudanese desert where people have had to travel 30 km. for water. A continuous supply is achieved by having two water-carrying camel teams, one of which travels each way each day. These are areas where it is difficult to find ground water by drilling and where even geophysical and seismic survey methods have little success. The Sudanese Rural Water and Development Corporation retained engineers experienced in water supply problems to help them achieve the aim of their "Freedom from Thirst" campaign. The method being pursued is to achieve local storage of the seasonal rainfall which is heavy, but which runs off rapidly to be lost in the desert. The main problem is to hold the water economically. The surface clay is often only 1–2 m. thick whereas a storage tank must be 8–9 m. deep if the water is to last the eight months of hot dry weather. The engineers have devised a method of excavating small village reservoirs and lining them with polythene. These reservoirs have a capacity of about 30,000 to 40,000 Mm^3. Termites proved a problem at first. They seek moisture and will burrow through polythene to reach it. So the "tanks" have to be triple lined, the outer two skins forming a sandwich filled with a gammexane slurry. Experimental reservoirs of this type have proved successful over several years and this "Third World" water supply project, which has attracted international support, is now expected to succeed where more sophisticated technology has proved too expensive.

The Department of Water and Development, Government of Cyprus, is also engaged in a number of major water resources projects. Late in 1975 the authority commissioned construction of a new 52 m. high dam across the Xeropotamus river at Asprokremmos in south west Cyprus. This dam which will store 50 Mm^3 of water to supply the 4700 ha. Paphos Irrigation Project, will be a clay-core gravel shell embankment. The irrigation system and services at Paphos are being built concurrently.

The list of new water management projects is continually growing and the result of all this activity has been the emergence of a new expertise which seeks to minimize the huge cost of exploiting new sources of water by combining the experience of geologists and hydrologists with those of specialist civil, hydraulic, chemical and mechanical engineers, in a discipline which has acquired the general title of water resources planning.

The world as a whole has learnt the lesson of New York in the 1965 drought. It has learnt that the underlying problem of delivering water where man needs it is no longer a problem of technology alone. Man has mastered the skills required and is capable of delivering water anywhere in the quantities and quality needed. Today the problem is a problem of planning—a problem of finding the money to pay for those skills and of planning so that the task is completed in time.

Notes to Present Edition

Costs

Since this text was written costs have of course escalated considerably: the cost of energy has more than quadrupled, which is a major factor in the adoption of desalination, and cement has almost matched energy in its price rises. As in all things in life the layman's laws of thermodynamics prevail—the First Law is "You don't get anything for nothing" and the second is "You get precious little for sixpence", which should now be amended to "You get precious little for 1 million pounds".

One way of keeping track of cost escalations is through the use of cost indices where a base index of 100 is taken at a fixed date and subsequent cost increases are scaled from this point. The figure opposite shows the composite plant construction cost index as compiled by the Journal Process Engineering for process plant. Using January 1970 = 100, the June 1976 index is 261.6, or an increase of 261 per cent in costs since 1970.

Projects conceived in the late 60s early 70s have to face the twin perils of cost escalation, as evidenced by the index for the appropriate industry, and an almost doubling of bank interest charges as well in the same period. It is little wonder then that sums of money many times greater than the original costs are bandied around for construction projects in the water industry. A typical cost escalation example for a reservoir is the Kielder Water (Northumberland) which is to use natural fill, a low-cost material; its 1972 cost of £10·3 million (for a yield to supply of

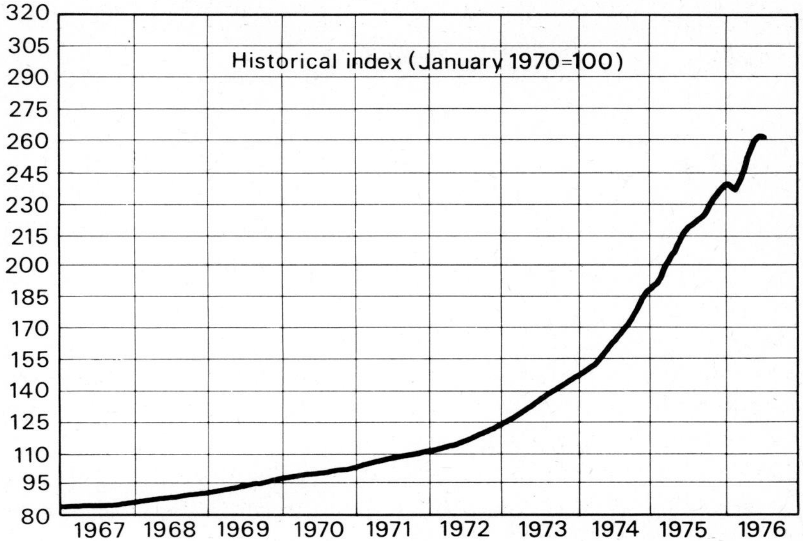

955 thousand cubic meters per day) is now estimated as £100 million by 1980 when the project is completed. Also, as depreciation charges are greater due to increased interest rates, the cost of water to the consumer will inevitably escalate. With this escalation the adoption of recycling techniques hitherto considered too costly will come to the fore so there is one consolation in that cost increases in the price of the basic commodity will lead to its being conserved—by no means a bad thing at that!

p. 111 The following continuation of the second paragraph amplifies the information on the efficiency of the Pelton wheel:

. . . wide variation in load, provided that the speed is constant. If the rotational speed of the turbine is raised or lowered from the optimum then the efficiency falls sharply. The optimum theoretical efficiency occurs when the bucket velocity is half that of the water jet velocity. In practice the maximum efficiency usually occurs at about 46/48 per cent of the jet velocity. Consequently although Pelton wheels are the most efficient of the three main types of water turbines they are less flexible, allowing only variation in torque while running at a constant speed. The direction of rotation of the Francis turbine (p. 113) is clockwise and the angle of the rotator blades should be almost 90° to the rotor blades.

p. 127 The aluminium industry is not in rapid growth now so the rest of the sentence and the whole of the next sentence should be ignored.

p. 154 Please skip the second part of the first sentence on this page . . . though a high CO_2 . . . and replace it with the following notes:

. . . in fact they frequently make the water safer to drink. Very soft water containing CO_2 will dissolve enough lead to render it unsafe, but in the presence of dissolved sulfates a protective layer of lead sulfate is built up on the inner surface of the pipe which considerably reduces the rate of attack. This layer can be seen as a white coating on the inside of old lead piping which has been used in hard water areas. In modern practice lead is not recommended for potable water if the hardness is less than approximately 150 p.p.m. (parts per million). Under these conditions copper or plastic piping (which are not susceptible to corrosion) should be used. These pipes also tend to be cheaper to buy and install than lead.

The dissolved salts of calcium, magnesium, zinc and iron are responsible for the "hardness" of water, although the last two rarely occur. These metals all give insoluble soaps which separate as a curd when contacted by normal washing soap (a mixture of the sodium salts of stearic, palmite and oleic acid):

$$\underset{\text{Washing Soap}}{2\,\text{Na (Soap)}} + \underset{\text{Soluble}}{\text{Ca}\,SO_4} \longrightarrow \overset{\text{Curd}}{\overset{\uparrow}{\text{Ca (Soap)}_2}} + \underset{\text{Soluble}}{Na_2\,SO_4}$$

The hardness salts are further designated as alkaline, or temporary, hardness and non-alkaline, or permanent, hardness.

The alkaline or temporary group consists only of the bicarbonates of the metals. However, only calcium bicarbonate is normally found in potable water. On heating the salt dissociates:

$$\underset{\text{Soluble}}{Ca\,(HCO)_3)_2} \xrightarrow{\text{heat}} \underset{\text{Insoluble}}{Ca\,CO_3\downarrow} + H_2O + CO_2\uparrow$$

giving a deposit on the heating surface (the "fur" inside a kettle). The non-alkaline or permanent group consists mainly of the sulfates and carbonates of the metals, together with occasional traces of chloride and nitrate. In modern water treatment technology the quantities present of these salts are corrected to their equivalent weight of calcium carbonate, i.e. the amount of calcium carbonate which would destroy the same weight of soap as would the salt being considered.

It must be realized from this that not all of the salts dissolved in a particular sample of water will necessarily give rise to hardness. The salts of metals which form soluble soaps will be excluded, these are normally only sodium and potassium. A sample taken from the tidal stretch of the River Mersey was found to have a total dissolved solids content of approximately 25,000 p.p.m. while the hardness salts were only present at 500 p.p.m. The large difference in these two values is largely accounted for by sodium chloride. In potable water the presence of sodium and potassium salts is usually very low so that for most practical purposes the hardness value of the water may be taken as the dissolved salt content.

p. 163 and 164 Please delete the sentence beginning at the bottom of p. 163 and continuing on p. 164 and substitute the following:

When an aluminium salt is dissolved in water some of it will ionize and react with the water ions:

$$Al_2(SO_4)_3 \rightleftharpoons 2[Al]^{3+} + 3(SO_4)^{2-}$$

$$H_2O \rightleftharpoons [H]^+ + [OH]^-$$

$$S[Al]^{3+} + 3[SO_4]^{2-} + [H]^+ + 6[OH]^- \rightarrow 2Al(OH)_3\downarrow + 3H_2SO_4$$

The aluminium hydroxide, being largely insoluble, precipitates as a floc leaving an acidic solution.

Any soluble aluminium salt could be used, but the cheapest is to be preferred. By cheapness is meant not the cost per kg., but the cost per unit weight of aluminium in the salt being used. In water treatment technology the salt normally used is loosely known as "alum", but it is not true alum, and is a special form of aluminium sulfate originally used by paper makers with less water of crystallization than normal aluminium sulfate.

Name	Formula	% Al by Weight
Papermakers Alum	$Al_2(SO_4)_3 . 14H_2O$	9.16
Aluminium sulfate	$Al_2(SO_4)_3 . 18H_2O$	8.06
Styptic, True or Barber's Alum	$K. Al(SO_4)_2 . 12H_2O$	5.74

The aluminium hydroxide $Al(OH)_3$ so formed in solution . . .

Suggested Reading

A. Bourgin *The Design of Dams* Pitman (London, 1953)

J. G. Brown (Ed.) *Hydro-electric Engineering Practice* 3 vols. Blackie (London and New York, 1958)

S. S. Butler *Engineering Hydrology* Prentice Hall (New Jersey, 1957)

Ven Te Chow (Ed.) *Handbook of Applied Hydrology* McGraw-Hill (New York, 1964)

I. E. Houk *Irrigation Engineering* Chapman and Hall (London, 1956)

P. C. G. Isaac *Public Health Engineering* E. & F. Spon (London, 1953) Barnes and Noble (New York, 1953)

O. W. Israelsen, V. E. Hansen *Irrigation Principles and Practices* John Wiley (New York, 1962)

P. H. Kuenen *Realms of Water* Cleaver-Hume Press (London, 1955) John Wiley (New York, 1956)

K. S. Spiegler *Principles of Desalination* Academic Press (New York, London, 1966)

N. P. Sporn *Fresh Water from Saline Waters* Pergamon Press (Oxford, 1966)

D. K. Todd *Ground Water Hydrology* John Wiley (New York, 1959) Chapman and Hall (London, 1959)

A. C. Twort *A Textbook of Water Supply* Edward Arnold (London, 1963) Elsevier (New York, 1964)

L. White, E. A. Prentis *Cofferdams* Columbia University Press (2nd Ed. New York, 1956)

Picture Credits

Page 8 Photo Ben Martin, *Time Magazine* © Time Inc.: 13 (Bottom left) Photo Dr. Georg Gerster, Zürich: 25 Photo Prof. C. Rathjens, Zentrale Farbbild Argentur G.m.b.H., Düsseldorf: 26 Photo Stella Snead: 31 Photo Paul Almasy: 32 Photo Stephen Harrison: 40 Photo Keystone Press Agency: 42 British Aeroplane Plastics Ltd., Bristol: 48 USDA Photo: 49 (Top) Press Information Department, Government of Pakistan, Rawalpindi (Bottom) Photo Paul Almasy: 52 Geological Museum, London: 57 Diana Wyllie Ltd., photo R. S. Scorer: 58 Hydrological Research Unit: 61 Geological Museum, London: 64 U.S. Geological Survey, photo M. F. Meier: 65 Raymond Thatcher (Studios) Ltd., Maidenhead: 68 Barnaby's/Ray Atkeson: 72 (Bottom left), 73 Picturepoint London: 77 (Bottom right) Photo Paul Almasy: 85 Embassy of Israel, London: 88 (Bottom left) Photo J. Allan Cash (Bottom right) Photo Paul Almasy: 89 Photo Zentrale Farbbild Argentur GmbH, Düsseldorf: 93 (Bottom) United Press International (U.K.) Ltd.: 97 (Top) Aero Service Corporation (Bottom left) South of Scotland Electricity Board (Bottom right) Photo Henri Germond, Lausanne: 101 Photo Paul Almasy: 105 (Right) Photos supplied by Sir Alexander Gibb & Partners: 108, 112, 113, 114, 115 The English Electric Company Limited: 122 (Top) Supplied by courtesy of the Central Electricity Generating Board (Bottom) The English Electric Company Limited: 123 Chloride Publicity Services: 129 Electricité de France, Paris: 132 Weir Westgarth Ltd., East Kilbride, Scotland: 136, 137 (Bottom) U.S. Geological Survey/Photo M. F. Meier: 140 (Bottom right) Photo Brad Messer, Houston: 141 (Bottom right) Photo United States Information Service, London: 144, 145 (Bottom right) United Kingdom Atomic Energy Authority: 149 (Bottom) Embassy of Israel, London: 150 Courtesy K. D. B. Johnson and to the Joint Symposium of BNES and BNF: 152 Photo Lennig Chemicals: 156 (Bottom left) Photo Prof. G. B. Winter: 156 (Bottom center & bottom right) Photos M. A. Young, M.Sc., B.D.S., Royal Dental Hospital, London: 157 (Bottom right) Water Resources Division of the U.S. Geological Survey: 159 Photo Ronald Toms: 160 Department of the Interior: Federal Water Pollution Control Administration, Washington: 173 (Bottom) Photos Lennig Chemicals: 176 Photo Dr. Georg Gerster, Zürich: 185 Photo British Iceberg Survey, London.

Index

Note: Numbers in italics refer to illustrations and captions to illustrations.